Gaylord High School
90 Livingston Blvd.
Gaylord, MI 49735

HEALTHY TEENS

Facing the Challenges of Young Lives

A Practical Guide for Parents, Caregivers, Educators, and Health Professionals

Third Edition

Alice R. McCarthy, Ph.D.

Bridge Communications, Inc.
Birmingham, Michigan

©2000 Alice R. McCarthy Ph.D. and Bridge Communications, Inc. This edition is an expansion and revision of a work previously published as *Healthy Teens: Success in High School and Beyond*, published by Bridge Communications, Inc., copyright ©1997 by Alice R. McCarthy.

Editors: Donna Raphael and David McCarthy
Researcher and Editor: Karen L. Kittredge
Illustrator: Mary Douse
Photographer: Michael Edward McCarthy
Stock Photography: Photodisc, Digital Vision
Designed by Ford & Earl Associates:
      Creative Director, Bonnie Detloff Zielinski
      Graphic Designer, M. Francheska Guerrero

Second Edition Writers and Editors: James H. McCarthy and Marcia Rayner Applegate

Library of Congress Catalog Card Number: 99-90976
ISBN 0-9621645-5-0
Printed in the U.S.A. on acid free recycled paper, 1999 ♻
Third Edition

Published and distributed by

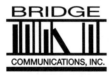

BRIDGE
COMMUNICATIONS, INC.

Books from Bridge Communications, Inc., are available at quantity discounts for educational use. For more information, write to Bridge Communications, Inc., 1450 Pilgrim Road, Birmingham, Michigan 48009, call 248-646-1020, fax 248-644-8546, or e-mail bridgecomm@aol.com. Web site: http://bridge-comm.com. Please send us your comments about *Healthy Teens,* Third Edition. Thank you.

I dedicate this book to my five children—Wally, David, Sharon, Jim, and Bill. You are grown up now and I am proud of you. Your support for my work has made a significant difference.

And to parents, caregivers, and professionals everywhere who are working with teens to promote a vision of a safe and healthy life for all adolescents within a context of teaching them responsibility, respect, honesty, justice and equality.

Contents

ACKNOWLEDGMENTS

The fear in writing acknowledgments rests with the author who forgets a special person or organization who has been begged to review his or her quote, or check the veracity of a set of statistics in 48 hours! And then there are authors who write "thanks to all those who have helped, and you know who you are." That is the easy way out. However, I am so grateful to many people for the assistance they have graciously given that I must try to mention as many as possible. *Healthy Teens* is stronger, based on their input and research.

The people who deserve every reader's thanks, and especially my own, are those who critiqued the second edition of *Healthy Teens* to ensure that the third edition would meet the needs of families across the nation. Busy, dedicated individuals completed a full reading of the second edition and answered a lengthy questionnaire. Included are Barbara Flis, parent of two adolescents; Donald Gainey, Ed.D., Principal, Milford High School, Massachusetts; Wanda Jubb, Ed.D., retired from the Centers for Disease Control and Prevention; Margaret Rose, M.S., Health Education Specialist, Utah State Office of Education; Jean Schultz, M.S., CHES, National Middle School Association; Victor Strasburger, MD, Chief, Division of Adolescent Medicine, Department of Pediatrics, University of New Mexico School of Medicine; Susan Wooley, Ph.D., Executive Director, American School Health Association; Paula R. Zaccone-Tzannetakis, Chair, Publications Committee, American Association for Health Education; Adam Uhlianuk, high school student; Harold Silk, M.A., Social Worker, Detroit School System; and Alex Braunstein, M.P.H., Research Associate, Health Management Research Center, University of Michigan, Ann Arbor.

I have conscientiously had the copy reviewed and the quotes approved, and in the process I have been amazed at the gracious responsiveness of scholars nationwide. I express appreciation to each of these professionals who assisted with reviews: David Rosen, MD, Craig Spangler, D.D.S., Steven Kempers, MD, W.J. McCarthy, MD (my son), Alexander Sackeyfio, MD, and J.P. Leleszi, D.O. Special thanks also to James Jaccard, Ph.D., who helped immeasurably in chapter four, and to Lloyd D. Johnston, Ph.D., whose work I have featured in all three editions of *Healthy Teens*. Likewise, Russell A. Barkley, Ph.D., Arthur L. Robin, Ph.D., and learning differences specialist Lou Stewart strengthened the copy in chapter three. Also, I called upon Amitai Etzioni, Ph.D., L. Rowell Huesmann, Ph.D., William Damon, Ph.D., and Peter Bearman, Ph.D., as I wrote about school violence. Steven J. Wolin, MD, and Sybil Wolin, Ph.D., checked the copy in chapter twelve on resiliency. A professional colleague from Lake Superior State University, William Munsell, graciously assisted as I rewrote material related to federal financial assistance.

Representatives from many publications gave permission to use outstanding material that I believe strengthen *Healthy Teens*. This included the *Weekly Reader 2® Magazine*; *The Bulletin* published by the National Association of Secondary School Principals; the Educational Development Center, Inc.; the *Prevention Researchers Newsletter*; and the Association for Supervision and Curriculum Development.

Others whose copy I received permission to print included the American Academy of Pediatrics; the National Clearinghouse on Families and Youth for Family and Youth Services Bureau; U.S. Department of Health and Human Services; The National PTA President Lois Jean White; The National Campaign to Prevent Teen Pregnancy; professionals from the Centers for Disease Control and Prevention (CDC); the U.S. Department of Education; Partnership for Family Involvement; and Drug Strategies' *Making the Grade: A Guide to School Drug Prevention*.

I give tremendous thanks to the expert counsel and review provided by five prestigious organizations and their representatives in the development of the current edition. Please refer to the facing page for a more detailed listing of their generous support.

Drawing on a long and positive experience with the Departments of Community Health and Education in Michigan, I am especially grateful for the continued support of Donald B. Sweeney, M.A.; Patricia Morgan, R.N., M.S.; Karen Petersmarck, Ph.D.; and Laurie Bechhofer, M.P.H. My longtime friend, health educator Barbara Bates, R.N., is always helpful with frank commentary.

Please refer to the list of contributors to the second edition of *Healthy Teens*, located in the back of the book. The foundation for the current edition was put in place with the help of these people who so willingly lent their expertise.

To my dedicated illustrator, Mary Douse, whose scores of careful, expressive drawings of young people in many moods well represent the essence of my work, I extend my grateful thanks. To Michael E. McCarthy, my talented 15-year-old grandson, who is now grown to the ripe old age of 16 during a year of writing, "thank you for your photos and your quiet modesty, courtesy, and patience toward your grandmother."

My editors—my son David N. McCarthy and also Donna Raphael—improved the clarity of the writing. Thank you. And thanks also to Laureen Motloch, who showed great patience in her diligent and superb keystroking work, and to Irene F. Thompson, graciously at the telephone daily about this book for over one year.

A very deep thank you goes to Karen Kittredge, M.S.W, M.Div. She is my talented and resourceful Web researcher who compiled and wrote many of our 500 annotations. She also edited as many as five rounds of readers of the twelve book chapters. This book would not have been as thorough or accurate without her scholarly help and support.

The design team from Ford & Earl Associates, Bonnie Detloff Zielinski and Francheska Guerrero, have shown amazing forbearance in working on a manuscript of this technical nature. They have designed a book that makes its author and the contributors very proud.

EXPERT COUNSEL AND REVIEW

The manuscript prepared for *Healthy Teens: Facing the Challenges of Young Lives*, Third Edition includes advanced and bold conceptualization of how the health of teens can be improved in the new millennium, through the support of families, schools, professionals, and institutions in society.

Throughout the manuscript preparation, Bridge Communications, Inc., has drawn on the research and advanced thinking of many distinguished scholars in the disciplines of adolescent development, education, and medicine. This is a book with many authors.

Bridge Communications, Inc., has also received expert counsel and review from professionals from five major national organizations:

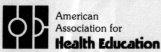

American Association for Health Education
Paula Zaccone-Tzannetakis, Ed.D., CHES
Chair, AAHE Publications Committee

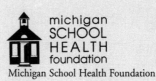

Michigan School Health Foundation

National Association of Secondary School Principals
Donald D. Gainey, Ed.D.
Principal, Milford High School, Massachusetts

National Middle School Association
Jean Schultz, M.S., CHES
Coordinator, Middle-Level AIDS
Prevention/Comprehensive Health Project

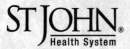

St. John Health System
Sylmara E. Chatman, M.D.
Medical Director, St. John Health System
School-Based Health Clinics

Alice R. McCarthy, Ph.D., Executive Editor and publisher of *Healthy Teens*, extends to these organizations, on behalf of teens and their families, her deep appreciation. She commends these organizations for their continuing service in advancing the health of young people. The views expressed in *Healthy Teens*, Third Edition, have not been approved by the governing or policy setting bodies of any of the above listed organizations and, accordingly, should not be construed as representing the policy of any of these organizations.

FOREWORD

All of us share a real concern about the many serious health risks that face our young people. Whether it is in our role as parents, educators, health providers or friends, we wonder what can be done to help youth negotiate these troubled times. An important key to protecting kids is the creation of a partnership between the school, the home, and the community to provide positive health messages. To be active partners in this protective circle we want to place around young people, parents and communities need current research, practical suggestions and down-to-earth advice. *Healthy Teens: Facing the Challenges of Young Lives* is a valuable resource to inform, educate and empower parents and other caring adults who are trying to make a meaningful contribution to protecting youth.

Alice R. McCarthy, Ph.D., the author of *Healthy Teens*, has a gift for presenting clear and compelling arguments for the vital role of citizen involvement in student health education programming. If you talk with this educator, she would convince you that a health education program that neglects the important roles of parents and the community is simply not going to be successful. She points out how important community involvement is in creating an effective health curriculum. She urges professionals to volunteer in health classes and adamantly advises schools to offer training, where necessary, to prepare adult volunteers. At the core of her ongoing work, she conveys the strong conviction that when parents and caregivers are taught to understand, in detail, the adverse consequences in young lives brought about by poor nutrition, lack of fitness, smoking, early sexual activity, substance abuse, violence, rape, abuse, harassment, along with depression and learning difficulties, then the parents will become the strongest advocates in the call to insist that comprehensive school health education be taught and valued.

Writing in the highly regarded book *Health Is Academic* (1998), David K. Lohrmann, Ph.D., and Susan F. Wooley, Ph.D., speak optimistically about the role of comprehensive health education, saying, ". . . [H]undreds of thousands of children and adolescents across the United States are becoming health literate through regular participation in school-based comprehensive health education." They add, ". . . these young people know how to avoid both health problems . . . such as unintentional injury due to car crashes or HIV infection and those that pose a greater threat during their adult years, such as cancer and heart disease."

Alice R. McCarthy, Ph.D. is also optimistic, noting that several large studies have found that high quality health education contributes to student knowledge, life skills, and positive health behaviors. While health educators engage in the important task of teaching skills to motivate students to improve their health, prevent disease, and reduce risk behaviors, Dr. McCarthy has produced thousands of pages of material over the years designed to help the families of children and youth understand the content and role of health education in students' lives. A recurring theme in her materials is to demonstrate and explain to adults the utmost importance of the family's role in student health education. Dr. McCarthy has the much needed ability to take complex yet vital health education research, and transform it into easy to use, approachable ideas and materials for the community. Evidence of this gift can be seen throughout her newsletters, books, curriculum materials, and in her creation of a very usable Family Resource Library bibliography for families.

In *Healthy Teens* Dr. McCarthy uses every persuasion, including the work of recent research findings and the words of strong leaders in health and education, to make her case: there is vital need for families to be deeply concerned about the health of their adolescents, and meeting this need is inseparable from supporting school health programming. We would be well advised to listen and learn.

Donald B. Sweeney, M.A.
Chief, School Health Unit
Michigan Department of Community Health

INTRODUCTION

This is a book about new ideas, ones that give structure to the dreams of one person to make a difference in the lives of children and youth ages eleven to eighteen today.

In 1995, I was called to try to explain to an esteemed group of colleagues why surveys from a carefully designed research project I had developed for parents had not emerged. I assured the group that the parents would reply to the surveys. All well and good, said the committee from a large metropolitan school district outside of Detroit, and yet a product was needed, since the activity was supported by a grant-funding source. A social worker in the group suggested I write some material about teens. An infant *Healthy Teens* was born. With that came positive reviews and wide distribution. (The surveys turned up weeks later—but that is another story!)

Project staff from the Michigan Model for Comprehensive School Health, representing many state-level departments, reviewed the booklet. They encouraged me to expand it into a book that would provide to adults vital health information about middle and secondary students. Thanks to this group's support, the first edition of *Healthy Teens* in 1996 sold out before it came off the press. In 1997, the second edition was published, with more expansive mental and physical health information; it was equally successful. The support of health professionals in Michigan is the prime reason why *Healthy Teens* has been widely accepted.

In developing this third edition, and moving to a national arena where I have fewer close professional colleagues in the health and education fields, I believed the second edition of *Healthy Teens* needed a complete review by eminent national authorities. I also wanted input from teens themselves. The individuals who assisted me in this comprehensive review are the real heroes in *Healthy Teens: Facing the Challenges of Young Lives*, Third Edition. They wrote passionately about what improvements were needed in book content and design.

With these reviews analyzed, I also believed that national organizations that cared about the health and welfare of young people would come on board to advise me and help me market the book once it was a reality. The Department of Education, Washington D.C. gave me assistance with referrals to national organizations. My plan was a comprehensive review of each chapter by a representative of the selected organizations. The experience of having six eminent professionals read and provide feedback on every word of every chapter was daunting at times. Even the logistics of having reviewers in every corner of the nation was difficult. I have only the highest praise for the reviewers, who took the time to offer detailed and thoughtful critiques of the material, with the singular motivation of helping children and youth. It quickly becomes clear that *Healthy Teens* is the product of many authors when one notes its comprehensiveness: the extensive annotated references and resources sections that include telephone and Web site listings, many selections of quotes from prominent researchers, and permissioned use of selections from dozens of nationally known organizations and writers.

While writing and rewriting to keep up with a difficult and thought-provoking year in the lives of teens and their families (1999), I drew inspiration from Bill Shore's book *The Cathedral Within* (Random House, 1999). Shore uses the cathedral as a metaphor to inspire visionaries who wish to create something that endures—like the cathedral builders of an earlier time did. He says, "Today there is another generation of Americans that desperately needs help: the generation who are poor, vulnerable and destined to repeat a familiar cycle of dysfunction and despair that is incongruous and unnecessary in prosperous America." Having given years of my life in community service, particularly to public schools and universities, I began to see a relationship between Shore's philosophy and my own. He says, "The great cathedrals did not soar skyward because their builders discovered new materials or financial resources; rather, the builders had a unique understanding of the human spirit that enabled them to use those materials in a new way." Perhaps my writing can serve to stem the despair of conscientious parents and caregivers, letting them know that their preteens and teens can reach adulthood well adjusted and well educated.

Perhaps these same adults will reach out to the children of whom Bill Shore speaks. They can do that effectively if they will take time to really listen to young people, to talk about issues of concern, and to advocate frequently for teens in schools and in the community. They can also make an important contribution by intervening against the destructive forces in the environment of all teens—such as the easy availability of tobacco, alcohol, and other drugs, thoughtless television programming, poor physical and mental health services for teens, and the neglect in our communities for teen involvement, meaningful work and community service. As Shore says:

> *History's defining moments are often born of crisis. But the unlikely genesis*
> *of today's defining moment is economic boom. Unemployment is*
> *at a twenty-four year low. Inflation barely exists. The stock market roars.*

America is at peace. If this is not the set of conditions under which our nation can and should mount a successful campaign to save the next generation of at-risk children, then I don't know what is.

Some authors recommend that certain chapters of their book be read when needed. Indeed, *Healthy Teens* invites that process in that much of the material is compartmentalized. However, there are themes not to be missed that run throughout the book: the need for a steady hand on the discipline rudder; a call for deep personal involvement in the interests of your child; the importance of giving kindly assurance and well-thought-out guidance throughout this growth period; a dedication to the strengthening of academic opportunity for all children in all schools—through volunteering and advocacy; the importance of continual vigilance to retain and strengthen health education and health programs centered in schools; and a need to recognize mental health issues for school staff and students and to advocate for improvement.

An important reason to read all twelve chapters is to be prepared beforehand for turning points in young lives, such as sexual maturation and the use of substances—tobacco, alcohol, and illegal drugs. Difficult societal circumstances also give good reason to read this material: the terrifying statistics of teen sexual abuse and sexual assault; the role of cliques, harassment, bullying, discrimination, and violence in a child's life; and the importance of the parent role in preventing early sexual intercourse, HIV/AIDS and other sexually transmitted diseases.

In chapter eleven, the guidelines for courses vital for middle schoolers and crucial national tests in high school are listed along with how to find financial aid for college and technical schools. This chapter is the result of my early academic work in vocational guidance. I believe strongly that the process of carefully choosing a field of work is of great significance in adult adjustment and happiness.

Read also to discover why you should speak up for all youngsters when health education programming is being challenged in your school, or how to organize when gangs and drug dealers move into your neighborhood. If your family life or your neighborhood environment seems far from perfect, read what resiliency (strength) experts say about children who do well in less than perfect circumstances.

"Build a cathedral," as Bill Shore says, or help me fulfill a dream that endures for the next generation. Please use the information in *Healthy Teens* to promote change for teens in your family, in your school, and in your community. For those with time, organizational skills, energy, and money, give freely so that all adolescents can move to adulthood with hope and courage.

Healthy Teens

Facing the Challenges of Young Lives

CHAPTER 1
HEALTHY BODIES, HEALTHY MINDS

Adolescence is a time of change—for your child and for you. Not only is your pre-teen or teen going through tremendous physical, emotional and developmental changes, but parents and guardians are finding they need to develop new ways of relating to their child. Some of the changes adolescents experience can seem frightening to themselves and to those who love them. Many times, the tools and techniques parents have used to interact with their child through the years suddenly seem as ineffective as ski poles in a canoe.

The goal of this newly revised and expanded third edition of *Healthy Teens* is to help adults understand their teens and guide them through the changes of the teenage years. It is written to give caring adults the knowledge they need to provide their growing children with love, support and guidance as they grow into adulthood.

The first chapter establishes the central themes—the healthy growth and development of the teens you care about. The chapter broadly defines adolescence, explains how growing up today differs from adolescent development a generation ago, and contains some general reminders for parents and caregivers about how to work with teens through early, middle, and late adolescence. The chapters that follow are more explicit, providing fuller details and information on various subjects related to teen health.

The following section of this chapter pp. 2-7 presents a slightly modified and updated version of the text that first appeared in *Supporting Your Adolescent: Tips for Parents*, produced by the National Clearinghouse on Families & Youth for the Family and Youth Services Bureau, U.S. Department of Health and Human Services. Within the section is information from the American Academy of Pediatrics, as noted in the text.

ADOLESCENCE

Adolescence is a time for young people to define their place in the family, peer groups, and the larger community. During this stage of their lives, young people struggle with the transition from childhood to adulthood. During childhood, they depended mainly on you, their parents and caregivers, for economic and emotional support and direction. In adulthood, though, they will be expected to achieve independence and make choices about school, work, and personal relationships that will affect every aspect of their future.

Without question, adolescence can be a difficult time for some young people. During this period, they must contend with physical changes, pressure to conform to current social trends and peer behaviors, and increased expectations from family members, teachers, and other adults. Adolescents also must deal with conflicting messages from parents, peers, or the media. They struggle with an increasing need to decide exactly how they "fit" in the society around them. Young people also feel pressure to perform academically or socially.

For some teens, the usual challenges of adolescence are compounded by difficult family situations, overcrowded classrooms, disintegrating neighborhoods, or exposure to alcohol or other drugs.

For some teens, the usual challenges of adolescence are compounded by difficult family situations, overcrowded classrooms, disintegrating neighborhoods, or exposure to alcohol or other drugs. Without support and guidance, these young people may fall victim to behaviors that place them, and others, at risk. In our society, those behaviors include dropping out of school, running away from home, joining gangs, using alcohol or drugs, or becoming involved in other law-breaking behaviors. Some youth may become depressed, leading to academic problems, social isolation, and/or self-destructive behavior.

Growing Up Today

Each generation of young people and their families face new, and perhaps more challenging, circumstances. Today, life for young people is characterized by increased family mobility, loss of extended family, and growing options with regard to careers, beliefs, and lifestyle choices. More transient lifestyles result in isolation from extended families and a breakdown in the feeling of community. There is a stronger presence of the media and entertainment in the lives of young people, coupled with the ever-expanding need to understand and be able to use new technology. Today, therefore, teens need greater self-direction and poise than ever before to successfully move from adolescence to adulthood.

Today's community and social structures place high demands on young people and their families. Fortunately, though, those systems also offer varied forms of support. Most communities have counseling services, specialized groups, hotlines, and educational courses for both youth and their parents. You will find many national hotlines listed in the reference and resource sections of this book. These organizations will help you to find referrals in your own community.

Helping your child move to independence requires that you understand healthy adolescent development and how to find the resources that can help you when your child gets off track. This book will help you understand teen development and find many resources to support the important work of keeping your young person mentally and physically healthy.

Tips for Parenting When Your Child Becomes an Adolescent

During adolescence, young people begin to take risks and experiment. They do so because they are moving from a family-centered world to the larger community within which they will begin to define their own identity. They may choose friends their parents do not approve of or try alcohol or other drugs. They may wear clothing that is trendy and in line with their peer group, begin comparing their families' lifestyles with those of other families, or break rules imposed by their parents or the larger community.

Through these actions, young people are testing the limits. They are recreating themselves in a fashion that they believe will allow them to survive without the day-to-day guidance of their parents. They also are trying to shift the balance of power and authority in their own direction. Parents and caregivers are understandably troubled by the confrontational nature of some adolescent behavior. Naturally, you also worry about other threats from the environment that may endanger the safety of your child, such as violent individuals, or the influence of their friends who smoke, drink or take drugs.

While there are no pat answers in parenting, the following strategies may help you support your child during adolescence while reducing the risk of serious harm to either your child or another person:

- EDUCATE YOURSELF ABOUT ADOLESCENT DEVELOPMENT. Learn about the behaviors to expect, the effects of physical changes, and ways to help your child deal with change.

The Academy of Pediatrics has this to say about the development of your teen:

In early adolescence (11-13 years), the physical changes of pubertal development signal dramatic and important milestones. Many young teens are concerned about whether their development is "normal" compared to their peers. With this concern about normality comes a preoccupation with one's appearance and a shift from parental and family activities to a stronger affiliation with peers. (See Table 1 on p. 11 for a description of developmental changes and psychosocial tasks of adolescence that may create stress within the family.)

The most useful tools in raising healthy young people are love, compassion, sensitivity, praise, understanding, and communication.

With middle adolescence (ages 14-16), peers assume even greater importance, and the drive for separation from parents (individuation) prompts teens to test the limits of parental control and authority. Parents may misinterpret a teen's increased need to affiliate with peers and establish a better sense of personal identity as a rejection of the family. In fact, most adolescents seek to maintain strong connections with their families, and most teens' values reflect those of their parents. However, conflict over control, if it is to occur, is most likely to begin and peak during middle adolescence. Independence can be an exciting prospect for the teen and a frightening thought for the parents. Normal behavior may be interpreted as outright rejection of the family, and conflicts over parental control often result.(See Table 1).

Ideally, late adolescence is characterized by a relatively stable identity, important mutual friendships, and a more adult relationship with parents. Most parents, including those who have experienced conflict with their teens, will find that the older adolescent has achieved a more stable equilibrium and can more easily balance family, peer/ friendship, and individual needs.

Reprinted with permission from the American Academy of Pediatrics. Helping Parents Communicate With Their Teens Part I: Assessment and General Strategies. Adolescent Health Update. 1999; 11(2).

- REMEMBER YOUR OWN ADOLESCENCE: YOUR CHANGING FEELINGS, ANGER AT AUTHORITY, AND FEARS AND HOPES. Look at your adolescent's behavior in context of those memories to help you keep perspective.

- THINK ABOUT TAKING A COURSE ON GOOD PARENTING. Parenting is a learned skill. Training can help even experienced parents by giving them new tools for supporting children through adolescence. Inquire at your school, your religious organization, the juvenile courts, and your PTA.

- LISTEN MORE THAN TALK. Young people have spent at least a decade as listeners in most situations. During adolescence, they want and need the chance to share their feelings and ideas and to begin recasting family beliefs, stories, and tradition in light of their changing identity. Review the section in this chapter on communication.

• TEACH YOUR ADOLESCENT ABOUT THE JOYS AND TROUBLES OF LIFE AND WAYS TO REVEL IN THE GOOD TIMES AND COPE WITH THE BAD. The myth that life is always easy or fair or that one should always be happy can lead to frustration for young people dealing with the realities of life.

• USE POSITIVE REINFORCEMENT FOR POSITIVE BEHAVIOR WHENEVER POSSIBLE; IT IS FAR MORE EFFECTIVE THAN CRITICISM OR PUNISHMENT FOR NEGATIVE BEHAVIOR. Words that belittle can hurt your adolescent's self-esteem. The most useful tools in raising healthy young people are love, compassion, sensitivity, praise, understanding, and communication. See the sections on problem-solving and being an authoritative parent/caregiver which follow later in this chapter.

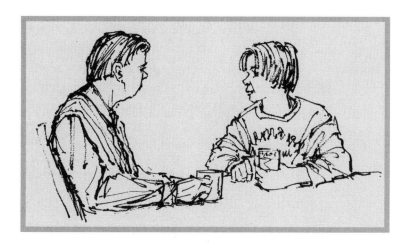

• TEACH YOUR ADOLESCENT THAT RIGHTS AND RESPONSIBILITIES GO HAND IN HAND, AND GIVE YOUR CHILD INCREASING RESPONSIBILITY FOR HIS OR HER PERSONAL WELL-BEING AND THAT OF THE FAMILY. Assist your child in finding opportunities to help at home, in the community, in the family business, and to become involved in family decision-making discussions. In doing so, seek your teen's input and help him or her to understand the process that you use to make those decisions. Look for situations that allow your child to test decision-making skills with the support of caring adults. Supportive adults can help provide your child with an understanding of the impact of those decisions on both your child and others. They also can assist your adolescent in coping with the results of these choices. Comprehensive health education programs lay a foundation for children and adolescents to practice decision-making. Support your school's efforts in this teaching. Review the curriculum being used and reinforce that teaching at home.

- HELP YOUR ADOLESCENT MOVE TOWARD INDEPENDENCE. For each young person, the need to assert independence will happen at different times and through different means. Becoming attuned to your children's attempts to operate independently will help you support those efforts and provide guidance when early attempts at decision-making result in less than desired outcomes. It is sometimes difficult for parents to give up control out of concern for their child's safety. Remember, though, that adolescents' skills in coping with increasing responsibility will be enhanced by parents' willingness to support them as they make choices and face new challenges.

- OFFER YOUR CHILD CHANCES TO BECOME INVOLVED IN THE COMMUNITY. All young people are searching to find their place in the world. Involving adolescents in developing solutions to community problems can shift their focus from themselves and help them develop skills and feel involved and empowered (see Chapter 12).

- SPEND QUALITY AND QUANTITY TIME WITH YOUR ADOLESCENT. Adolescence is a time when young people naturally begin to pull away from the family and spend more time at school, with friends, or at a job. Research tells us that time spent with caring parents and other adults is key to young people's ability to grow emotionally and socially. Take advantage of times that your adolescent is home, over dinner, in the car, or watching a ball game, to continue building your relationship. Become

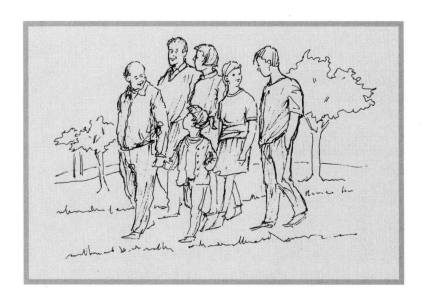

involved in your child's outside interests. Your involvement will show your support and help you stay informed about your child's life.

- ENCOURAGE OTHER CARING ADULTS, INCLUDING FRIENDS AND RELATIVES, TO SPEND TIME WITH YOUR ADOLESCENT. Aunts and uncles, adult neighbors, and work associates can offer your teen further support, guidance, and attention. These people can often mentor your child during both easy and difficult times in adolescence.

- ACCEPT THAT YOU HAVE FEELINGS TOO. You may feel frustrated, angry, or sad during difficult times with your adolescent. Being a good parent or caregiver doesn't mean being perfect. Model the ability to apologize when you feel that you let your emotions get the best of you. Your example will help your child understand human frailty and ways of mending relationships strained by stress or disagreement.

- SEEK SUPPORT AND GUIDANCE FOR YOURSELF IN DEALING WITH THE CHANGES IN A CHILD MOVING THROUGH ADOLESCENCE. Learn about the signs of crisis, and talk with other parents or professionals. By doing so, you can begin to tell the difference between adolescent behavior that indicates your teen is in crisis and the usual behavior associated with developing teens. This book outlines behaviors that will help you notice if life is not going well for your teen. Especially note Chapters 3-10 if you are seeking help in these areas.

- REMEMBER THAT MOST YOUTH HAVE PROBLEMS AT SOME TIME. Acting-out behavior can be a normal part of becoming an adult. Parents and caregivers sometimes needlessly feel embarrassed when their child is having trouble. Do not assume that your child's behavior always reflects on the quality of your parenting. Please know that many competent professionals, especially at your teen's school, stand ready to help or make referrals in times of stress.

- DO NOT ALWAYS PUSH FOR DRASTIC SOLUTIONS. Sometimes young people just need time and support to work through their problems.

- CONTINUE TO PROVIDE YOUR ADOLESCENT WITH POSITIVE FEEDBACK AND OPPORTUNITIES TO GROW. Reflect on what you want for your children: health, happiness, and movement toward a promising future. Offer them chances to strengthen their skills and develop a sense of competence, usefulness, and belonging.

COMMUNICATING WITH YOUR TEEN

Talk with your teen? Having a heart-to-heart with an outer space alien may seem easier. But parent-teen communication doesn't have to be stressful, strained or a challenge.

Sure, teenagers may argue nearly every point their parent or caregiver makes. They may question the logic of adults, or they even may clam up with Mom and Dad, while chatting endlessly with friends.

That simply means they're exercising their thinking skills, flexing their cognitive muscles, as they struggle toward independence and to crystallize their own identity. Keep in mind that no matter how eagerly teens appear to distance themselves from family, they need and want parental love and support—even if they don't admit it.

Loving, caring communication that says "I'm here for you," even when your teen says "leave me alone," is rooted in a good rapport between parent and adolescent. Healthy communication goes beyond dinner table chat or a quick exchange in the car on the way to school. It's an ongoing process that may include everything from watching movies together to discussing politics and values. Parents have a better chance of influencing their teen's choices if they "connect" with their child on a daily basis. And they'll tackle serious subjects more easily if they routinely discuss non-threatening topics with their children.

But parents and caregivers also need to recognize that communication occurs in many forms. It doesn't always fit neatly into a discussion or a trek to the movies. Teens continuously send messages, whether through sulky silences, a slammed door or a warm hug. Adults must learn to translate non-verbal "talk" and physical cues.

If your teen doesn't want to talk, you can break the ice by asking questions that focus on personal interests. Teens often enjoy talking about themselves, family matters, current affairs, the future, and emotional issues. Talk about their interests and share your own feelings. Ask questions that will provoke more than one-word answers. Or ask your teen to "tell me more."

Some teens are more likely to "open up" while engaged in an activity than simply when talking one-on-one. Consider planning an outing or sharing an activity or hobby to help jump-start conversation. Ask your teen if it's a good time to talk. If not, pinpoint a better time and be sure to keep the "appointment."

Try to remain approachable, no matter what the subject is and look for "teachable mo-

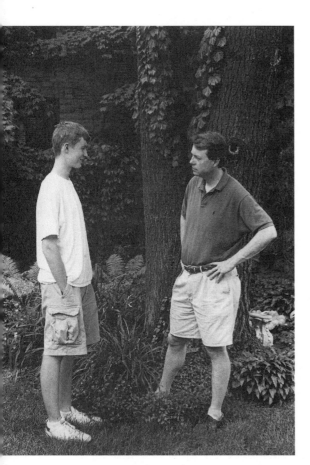

"Tell me more about what happened last night."

ments" in daily activities and through the media. You will find support and help for talking to your teen in the chapters that follow.

Please remember that criticism, ridicule, too much advice and a disregard for your teen's problems create roadblocks to communication. Treating your teen with respect, showing love and appreciation and pointing out strengths, can keep lines of communication open.

Becoming a Good Listener
Building rapport and genuine communication begins with listening:

- Pay attention. Establish eye contact.
- Do not interrupt or finish your teen's sentences. Try not to force your opinions on your teen.
- Rephrase your teen's comments in your own words to show that you understand. Give non-verbal encouragement.
- Do not become defensive if your teen criticizes you.

Try Problem-Solving

Collaborative problem-solving, such as is taught in health education classes, can help parents and teens resolve differences and minimize hostility. After establishing ground rules, each side explains their view of the issue. They brainstorm solutions and discuss options. A written agreement and follow-up discussion can help resolve disagreements. Teach your sons and your daughters how to handle anger, jealousy and sadness—and how to manage disappointment, rejection, ridicule, exclusion and conflict. Talk about how you manage and model positive behavior just as often as you have the chance. You'll do this mostly by how you behave.

Parents may want to consider these additional tips for communicating with girls:

- Talk to your daughter about gender-based discrimination. Teach her to identify specific ways in which institutions and individuals may treat her as inferior just based on her being a woman, and how she can cope with this. Make her aware that national legislation was passed specifically to address gender inequity in school systems (Title IX, See Table 2, Gains for Women.)
- Encourage your daughter to keep a journal. This will help her to define her goals and pinpoint her progress.

- Help her gather information about real world occupations that interest her.
- Build her up when she tears herself down. Studies show that girls are more likely to blame themselves rather than circumstances when things go wrong.
- Encourage her involvement in organized sports and activities.
- Find mentors and role models for your daughter.

Parents can consider these tips for communicating with boys:

- Teach your son empathy. Develop emotional solidarity between you and your son by showing tenderness.
- Talk to your son about gender-based discrimination. Teach him to treat all women and girls with dignity and respect, and how to cope with others around him who are not doing this. Make him aware that national legislation was passed specifically to address gender inequity in school systems (Title IX).
- Teach, by example, empathy, kindness, and caring.
- Gather information about occupations that interest him. Appreciate that your son may have different interests than you do. Try to involve yourself in your son's interests.
- Find mentors and role models for your son.

Being an Authoritative Parent

Good communication keeps parents and teens connected. Parents who set clear expectations and achievement standards for behavior, enforce rules consistently and respect their teen, demonstrate authoritative parenting. Tips to keep in mind:

1. Reassure your teen with your love and trust.

2. Know when to be flexible and when to stand your ground on an issue.

3. Be willing to re-evaluate rules.

Table 1: Adolescent Developmental Needs and Expected Behaviors

Developmental Needs	How Teens May See It	How Parents May See It	Solutions
Independence, autonomy, and individuation	Parents are too controlling, not giving enough freedom	Teen constantly challenging the "order of command"	Negotiate rules together
	Teen doesn't have enough input into rules, household responsibilities	Teen wants to be able to "call the shots"	Link increased independence to increased responsibilities
		Teen doesn't want to follow rules, or meet responsibilities	Provide safe opportunities for exploration/freedom
		Teen wants more freedom, challenges any restriction	Maintain high expectations, allow some rebellion, but set limits and enforce rules consistently
		Often ambivalent, erratic, moody	
Peer Affiliation	Wants to spend more time with friends, less time with family	Teen rejects family to be with friend	Allow teen time to develop important friendships
		Embarrassed to be seen with family	Establish family rituals and make it clear that teen is expected to participate
			Allow teen freedom to choose friends
Identity Formation	Needs to "try on" and experiment with a lot of different identities	Egocentric, narcissistic, and inconsistent	Be patient
			Keep sense of humor
			Choose your battles
	Needs privacy and space	Secretive	Respect need for privacy, but be aware that too much seclusion may be a sign of problems

Table continues on the next page.

Table 1: Adolescent Developmental Needs and Expected Behaviors (Cont.)

Developmental Needs	How Teens May See It	How Parents May See It	Solutions
Cognitive Development	Teen can think for himself	Argumentative	Provide rationale for decisions
	Can reason abstractly	Challenging	Appreciate intellectual development as positive change
		Teen (knows it all)	
		Opinionated	Remember that judgement and insight are limited

Reprinted with permission from the American Academy of Pediatrics. Helping Parents Communicate With Their Teens Part I: Assessment and General Strategies. Adolescent Health Update. 1999; 11(2): 3.

Table 2: Title IX, Gains for Women

Women have made great strides in participation and ownership in the nearly three decades Title IX has been in effect. Some key areas:

Girls in High School Sports

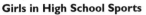
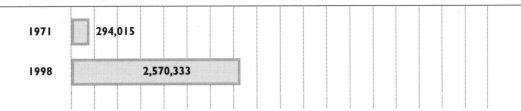

1971 — 294,015
1998 — 2,570,333

Women Doctors

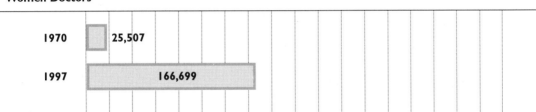

1970 — 25,507
1997 — 166,699

Women Participating in Workforce

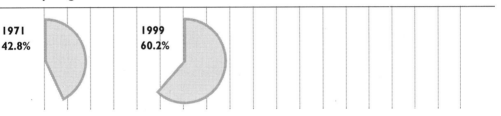

1971
42.8%

1999
60.2%

Woman-owned Businesses

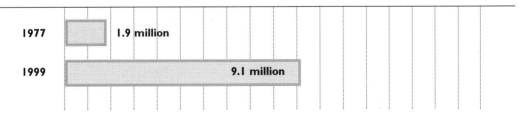

1977 — 1.9 million
1999 — 9.1 million

Reprinted with permission from the *Detroit Free Press*, 7/9/99, "Girls ride Title IX to success as women."

REFERENCES AND RESOURCES   R/R

Before It's Too Late: Why Some Kids Get Into Trouble and What Parents Can Do About It, Stanton E. Samenow (Times Books, 1999, $24.00). In this newly revised and expanded edition of the classic guide, clinical psychologist Stanton Samenow discusses the difficult subject of "problem children" with compassion, reassurance, and welcome clarity. Offers practical suggestions for taking action now.

Caring for Your Adolescent, Ages 12-21 (The American Academy of Pediatrics: Division of Publications, 141 Northwest Point Blvd., P.O. Box 927, Elk Grove Village, IL, 60009-0927, 800-433-9016, 1992, $19.95). Editorial direction by a distinguished pediatrician; contributions by 30 specialists in adolescent medicine. It is a comprehensive book written in a humane tone. Complete reference guide to developmental stages and issues facing adolescents, giving detailed coverage of specific problems such as depression, suicide, substance abuse, AIDS and other sexually transmitted diseases, learning disorders, intensive sports training, obesity and eating disorders, common illnesses and infections. Highly recommended.

Discipline: A Sourcebook of 50 Failsafe Techniques for Parents, James Windell (Collier Books, 1991, $12.95). A psychologist for the juvenile court offers practical tips for parents to build self-control in children of all ages.

Effective Black Parenting: A Review and Synthesis of Black Perspectives, Kerby T. Alvy, Ph.D. (available through the Center for Improvement of Child Caring, Studio City, California, 800-325-CICC, $14.95). A complete profile of effective parenting for African-American families, based on what African-American scholars like James Comer and Alvin Poussaint believe are the most important issues and challenges in this area.

Emotional Intelligence, Daniel Goleman (Bantam Books, 1997, $13.95). Fascinating and challenging book grounded in recent scientific research. Not an easy read, but well worth the effort. Emotional intelligence includes self-awareness, impulse control, diligence, social skills, and empathy.

Every Family Needs a C.E.O., Reuben Bar-Levav (Fatherling Inc. Press, 1995, $19.95). A psychiatrist for 30 years is encouraging to parents, stating clearly that in order to raise responsible children, there must be a person in charge. A manual full of practical solutions, this volume shows that raising sensible youngsters is a difficult task, but that it can be done.

Failing at Fairness: How Our Schools Cheat Girls, Myra and David Sadker (Touchstone Press, 1995, $12.00). Report of a definitive study that brings attention to how schools are not meeting the needs of girls and young women. Very important for awareness and planning for change.

Family Life and School Achievement: Why Poor Black Children Succeed or Fail, Reginald M. Clark (University of Chicago Press, 1984, $9.95). Compares the backgrounds of high achieving inner city teenagers with peers who are failing, and determines what makes the difference.

Finding Our Way: The Teen Girls' Survival Guide, Allison Abner and Linda Villarosa (HarperPerennial, 1996, $13.50). Written by a freelance journalist and the executive editor of *Essence* magazine, both African Americans, this candid book covers most of the important subjects—body image, puberty, sexual development, relationships with friends and family, nutrition, discussion of tattoos and plastic surgery, and personal safety. Judiciously used comments from teens personalize the reading, and there's an obvious attempt to encompass multicultural difference. The chapter on body image, for example, notes differences in the "ideal" body type as accepted by African Americans and by whites.

Get it? Got it. Good!: A Guide for Teenagers, Carol Noël, ed. (Serious Business, Inc., 1996, $7.95). This outstanding book for teens covers self esteem, college, working, depression, decision-making, sex, AIDS, healthy eating, crime, alcohol, smoking, and substance abuse.

Get Out of My Life, But First Could You Drive Me and Cheryl to the Mall?: A Parent's Guide to the New Teenager, Anthony E. Wolf (The Noonday Press, 1992, $11.00). About adolescence—explained with quotes from kids and their families, and chapters on what they do and why, and a multitude of other issues of great concern to adults with teens. All written with humor.

Grounded for Life?!: Stop Blowing Your Fuse and Start Communicating With Your Teenager, Louise Felton Tracy (Parenting Press, Inc., 1994, $12.95). Chapters include: Begin by Changing Yourself, Natural Consequences, Parent-Owned Problems, Love in Action, Resistance and Acceptance, Understanding Teen Sexuality, Parental Persistence.

Growing Up Adopted, Peter L. Benson, Dr. Anu Sharma, and Eugene C. Roehlkepartain (Search Institute, 1995, 800-888-7828, $7.95). Detailed information on the findings of Search Institute's study of adopted teens and their families.

How Schools Shortchange Girls: The AAUW Report: A Study of Major Findings on Girls and Education (Marlowe & Co., 1995, $12.95). The American Association of University Women's 1992 landmark study on girls and education. A volume based on more than 1,300 studies challenges common assumptions that girls are treated equally in public schools. Call the AAUW at 800-225-9998 x421 for the updated version from May 1998.

How to Develop Self-Esteem in Your Child: 6 Vital Ingredients, Bettie B. Youngs (Columbine Trade, 1993, $10.00). A leading educator presents a step-by-step handbook for parents to help build strong positive self-esteem.

Life on the Edge: A Young Adult's Guide to a Meaningful Future, James C. Dobson (Word Books, 1995, $19.99). For older adolescents (ages 16-26) and their parents, Dobson suggests ways to approach the life-altering decisions of college, marriage, and family.

Living With a Work in Progress: A Parents' Guide to Surviving Adolescence, Carol G. Freeman (National Middle School Association, 1996, $12.00). Laugh a lot and learn a lot from this attractive resource for parents. Written by a mother of young adolescents, this book provides true-to-life anecdotes organized into such sections as Uncommon Traits: Snits, Zits, and Flammable Hair, and Schoolwork: Choosing Your Battles. Specific articles deal with a range of topics including saying "no," telephones, stereotyping, the report card, and rejection.

Making Sense of Your Teenager, Lawrence Kutner (William Morrow, 1997, $11.00). Kutner emphasizes communication, limit setting, and freedom of expression as keys to a healthy parent-teen relationship. He shows practical ways to apply these ideas in your day-to-day interactions with your teen. Discussion of serious issues such as depression, eating disorders, and sexuality helps parents steer a sane and sensible path. The author's deft humor makes his anecdotes and examples inspiring and down-to-earth. He is very solid in his advice.

New Moon Network: For Adults Who Care About Girls, (New Moon Publishing, PO Box 3620, Columbus Ave, Duluth MN 55803-3620. E-mail address: newmoon@computerpro.com. Web site: www. newmoon.org). This bi-monthly black and white 16-page publication offers amazing insights into the world that adolescent girls populate today, including issues like menstruation, popularity, sexuality, self-image and responsibility. New Moon also publishes a companion magazine for girls ages 8-14 called *New Moon: The Magazine for Girls and Their Dreams*, which is written by teenage girls and contains stories, fiction, poetry, interviews, experiments, heroes and more.

The Parenting TightRope: A Flexible Approach to Building Self-Esteem, Julie Stitt (Momentum Books, 1994, $9.95). Stitt, the prevention specialist at Common Ground, a leading crisis center in Michigan, bases her book on experience with teens.

Parenting With a Purpose: A Positive Approach for Raising Confident, Caring Youth, Dean Feldmeyer and Eugene C. Roehlkepartain (Search Institute, 1995, free, 800-888-7828). 14-page, full-color booklet on ways families can build assets in young people. Positive and inspiring.

Parents and Adolescents Living Together, Part 1: The Basics, and *Parents and Adolescents Living Together, Part 2: Family Problem Solving*, Gerald Patterson and Marion Forgatch (Castalia Publishing, 1987, Part 1: $12.95, Part 2: $13.95). Part 1: Step-by-step approach to handling arguments and conflicts between parents and teens. Part 2: Negotiation skills for resolving difficult issues.

Peer Pressure Reversal: An Adult Guide to Developing a Responsible Child, Sharon Scott (Human Resource Development Press, 1997, $14.95). Provides parents with a step-by-step approach to teaching how to handle peer pressure.

Positive Discipline for Teenagers: Resolving Conflict With Your Teenage Son or Daughter, Lynn Lott and Jane Nelsen (Prima Publishing, 1994, $14.95). This book describes individuation, the process of establishing a separate identity, which every teen must go through to reach his or her full potential. It shares how parents can get cooperation from their children without threats.

Raising A Son: Parents and the Making of a Healthy Man, Don Elium and Jeanne Elium (Celestial Arts, 1996, $12.95). This guide to raising a male child describes the hidden problems of boy-specific needs. It stresses the importance of the father's role in a son's development, and answers questions about male aggression, hostility, violence, and sexuality. Excellent bibliography included.

Raising Boys: Why Boys Are Different—And How to Help Them Become Happy and Well-Balanced Men, Steve Biddulph (Celestial Arts, 1998, $12.95). Includes lots of information about boy development in an entertaining and easy-to-read format. Gives tips on communication as well as other topics, including bullying, discipline and role models. Relates developmental needs to school and parenting.

Real Boys: Rescuing Our Sons from the Myths of Boyhood, William Pollack (Owl Books, 1999, $13.95). This book is written by a clinical psychologist and co-director of the Center for Men at McLean Hospital/Harvard Medical School. Based on nearly 20 years of clinical experience with boys, the author conveys the message that boys, struggling under the weight of outdated gender stereotypes, are in trouble. He dismantles commonplace myths of boyhood, and discusses how to help boys to break free from the "boy code." He deals with the most serious consequences of this code, including depression and violence, and concludes the book by putting forth a revised code for boys to live by.

Rebel Without A Car: Surviving and Appreciating Your Child's Teen Years, Fred Mednick (Fairview Press, 1996, $12.95). This book, written by a high school principal (and father of two), covers adolescence with humor, practical tips and believable examples. Topics include teens and behavior, morality, sexuality, school, girls, gay teens and motivation. Parents and grandparents alike will relate.

Reviving Ophelia: Saving the Selves of Adolescent Girls, Mary Pipher (Ballantine Books, 1995, $14.00). The author/therapist describes the process through which many teenage girls lose spark, interest, and even IQ points as a "girl-poisoning" society forces a choice between being shunned for staying true to oneself and struggling to stay within a narrow definition of female. She offers prescriptions for changing society and helping girls resist.

The Roller-Coaster Years: Raising Your Child Through the Maddening Yet Magical Middle School Years, Charlene C. Giannetti and Margaret Sagarese (Broadway Books, 1997, $15.00). For the 20 million parents of 10-15 year-olds, this book is a guide to mastering the ups and downs of early adolescence. Drawing together the latest information from experts, supported and advised by the National Middle School Association, and with surprising insights from the authors' own surveys of parents, teachers, and the children themselves, *The Roller Coaster Years* covers every facet of the physical, social, emotional, and intellectual development of early adolescents. These include: appearance anxiety, distractibility, fears and other emotions, the battle for independence, sibling rivalry, success in school, friendship and peer pressure, sexual awakening, the lure of tobacco, drugs, and alcohol, the promise and peril of electronic media, and sticky questions about your own past. Highly recommended.

Safeguarding Your Teenager From the Dragons of Life: A Parent's Guide to the Adolescent Years, Bettie B. Youngs (Health Communications Inc., 1993, $11.95). This guide offers insights designed to help parents understand the world teenagers live in, highlighting developmental stages for each age group (including intellectual, physical, psychological, social, moral, and ethical stages).

The 7 Habits of Highly Effective Families, Stephin R. Covey (Golden Seal Books, 1997, $25.00). Stephen R. Covey is well known especially for his book *The 7 Habits of Highly Effective People*. He says, however, that this book has been his most passionate project. The author and his wife have nine children, and many of their own family stories are described in this book.

Smart Girls: A New Psychology of Girls, Women and Giftedness, Barbara A. Kerr (Gifted Psychology Press, 1997, $24.00). Why do talented, gifted girls so often fail to realize their potential as they reach adolescence and adulthood? This outstanding book summarizes research on gifted girls, presents biographies of eminent women and examines the current educational and family milieu.

Strong Mothers, Strong Sons, Ann P. Caron (HarperPerrenial, 1995, $14.00). A book for mothers that focuses on the special needs of male adolescents, including the conflict of violence vs. sensitivity, athletics, sexuality, and attitudes toward women.

Supporting Your Adolescent: Tips for Parents, August 1996 (National Clearinghouse on Families & Youth for the Family Youth Services Bureau, U.S. Dept of Health and Human Services. Web site: www.ncfy.com/supporti.htm). See the first seven pages of this chapter's text, which uses significant sections of this very helpful report.

Things Will Be Different for My Daughter: A Practical Guide to Building Her Self-Esteem and Self-Reliance, Mindy Bingham (Penguin USA, 1995, $15.95). Handbook to help parents build their daughter's self-esteem throughout each stage of her life by confronting traditional challenges to her success and suggesting ways to overcome them.

The Working Parents Help Book: Practical Advice for Dealing With the Day-to-Day Challenges of Kids and Careers, Susan Crites Price and Tom Price (Petersons Guides, 1996, $16.95). The classic guide for working parents everywhere. A 1994 Parents Choice Award winner (includes windows Working Parents Helpware®).

You and Your Adolescent: A Parent's Guide for Ages 10-20, Laurence Steinberg and Ann Levine (HarperCollins, 1997, $15.00). This book will help you understand: family communication and problem-solving; the physical and emotional changes of puberty; intellectual and moral growth; cliques and crowds, popularity, and peer pressure; sex and the high school student; myths and facts about cigarettes, alcohol, and drugs; how teenagers think; and the transition to adulthood. This is a calm, measured book filled with thoughtful advice. Highly recommended.

Your Child's Growing Mind: A Guide to Learning and Brain Development from Birth to Adolescence, Jane M. Healy (Main Street Books, 1994, $13.95). This book became an instant classic when it was published in 1987, and has been a cornerstone for educators ever since. Now revised and updated to reflect recent findings in brain research, this book guides parents, teachers, and caregivers as they gauge the level of development of an individual child's brain.

Chapter 2
Teens, Families, and Schools

This chapter makes a poignant, yet logical plea for parents and caregivers, both as family and community members, to join with school administrators and teachers in planning for ways to be involved in the school life of their pre-teens and teens. In keeping with the themes of this book, a research-based explanation and specific suggestions are offered for the great value of having the family involved in school health education.

Family Involvement in Health Education

As teens, families, and schools move into the third millennium, there is even more compelling evidence that a strong family-school partnership can make a difference in teen school success. Studies have shown for some time that family involvement in the school life of their teens means higher grades, test scores, graduation rates, and college attendance. Now a national study of 90,000 young people and their families, The National Longitudinal Study of Adolescent Health (Add Health Study) indicates that families and schools make a significant difference in the life of their adolescent in additional ways.

The most critical threats to adolescent health arise from risky behaviors. Immediate, and potentially life-threatening, health risks come about because teens use alcohol and other drugs, have early and unprotected sex, and are exposed to or participate in violent situations such as being threatened or injured with a weapon. Driving under the influence of alcohol or drugs is high-risk behavior. Long-term health consequences can occur from smoking cigarettes, eating a poor diet, or leading a physically inactive life style. To counterbalance that information, the Add Health study shows that a bulwark against these health threats is the protection that comes to a teen who feels connected with parents, family, and school. When parents have high expectations for school performance, and are physically present in the home at key times, children are more likely to be protected from involvement in behaviors that can damage them. The study also showed that students who feel attached to their family report lower levels of being emotionally upset. They are less likely to think about, or attempt, suicide, to engage in violent behavior or smoke cigarettes, drink alcohol or use marijuana, and more likely to delay first intercourse when they feel a connection with their family or school.

> Family involvement in the school life of their teens means higher grades, test scores, graduation rates, and college attendance.

How can we build the web between family and schools so that success for more teens is ensured? One important strand in that web is parents who take an active role in health education at their children's schools. In a 1999 survey, respondents ranked health education higher than math, language arts, science, and history, when asked what students should know by the time they graduate from high school. The research that details these surprising findings comes from *What Americans Believe Students Should Know: A Survey of Young Adults.* Listed below are the health education standards about which the Gallup poll surveyed Americans:

- Understands aspects of substance use and abuse.
- Understands the relationship of family health to individual health.
- Knows essential concepts about the prevention and control of disease.
- Knows how to maintain mental and emotional health.
- Knows the availability and effective use of health services, products, and information.
- Understands essential concepts about nutrition and diet.
- Knows essential concepts and practices concerning injury prevention and safety.
- Understands the fundamental aspects of growth and development.
- Knows how to maintain and promote personal health.
- Knows environmental and outside factors that affect individual and community health.

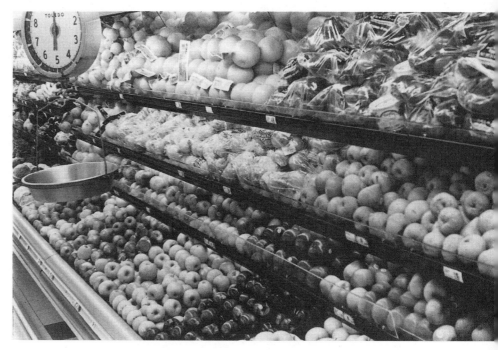

Americans want students to understand the essential concepts of nutrition and diet—such as eating many fruits and vegetables daily.

Nine of the 10 health education standards listed here appeared in the top 25 standards chosen overall, and the majority of respondents rated all 10 health standards as "definitely" needing to be included in the curriculum. Parents, caregivers, and community health professionals can use this information as they work with school administrators and school boards to advocate for health education. Parents, caregivers, and professionals can make a real difference in the lives of teens by advocating that their schools teach lessons focusing on these standards.

Reporting in the November 1998 issue of the *Bulletin*, published by the National Association of Secondary School Principals (NASSP), authors Susan Wooley, Eva Marx, and Becky Smith have this to say:

> *While few dispute that students' physical, mental, emotional, and social health plays a role in how well they learn, the time allocated for students to acquire the information and skills they need to make appropriate decisions about their health is often minimal. Although most secondary schools do require some health instruction, this usually consists of one semester in high school and one at the middle level. In most U.S. schools, the person teaching the health class has no academic training in the subject.*

In some schools, health classes are relegated to the cafeteria or gymnasium. Such decisions communicate to students and the faculty how little administrators value health issues.

SETTING PRIORITIES

. . . First, determine your students' priority needs for health information and skills. Data are probably available from sources such as the school nurse, attendance records, and discipline reports. Local juvenile officers, medical care providers in the community, or anonymous surveys of students can provide information about the types of activities youth engage in that put them at risk for poor attendance or academic performance. . . .

Addressing problems adequately requires sufficient time. In one study, researchers found it took 15 instructional hours to change students' understanding and 45 hours to change behavior. . . . Anyone who expects to reduce teen pregnancy, for instance, through one or two classroom periods of instruction will be disappointed.

There are National Health Education Standards that have changed the focus of health education from content and concepts to skills and competencies. Health literacy, the focus of the standards, is "the capacity of individuals to obtain, interpret, and understand basic health information and services and the competence to use such information and services in ways which enhance health."

The standards can inform decisions about curricula that will enhance students' health literacy. These standards, which are compatible with the National Education Goals 2000, are:

- *Students will comprehend concepts related to health promotion and disease prevention.*
- *Students will demonstrate the ability to access valid health information and health-promoting products and services.*
- *Students will demonstrate the ability to practice health-enhancing behaviors and reduce health risks.*
- *Students will analyze the influence of culture, media, technology, and other factors on health.*
- *Students will demonstrate the ability to use interpersonal communication skills to enhance health.*
- *Students will demonstrate the ability to use goal-setting and decision-making skills to enhance health.*
- *Students will demonstrate the ability to advocate for personal, family, and community health.*

Building on and linked to the National Health Education Standards are state interpretations of those standards. The Council of Chief State School Officers has developed student assessments in health education. A CD-ROM, available in participating states, includes selected responses and constructed response items as well as performance tasks and events. It also includes scoring rubrics. More than half of all states currently participate in a health education assessment project known as Assessing Health Literacy. *To find out whether your state has access to the assessment items, contact the health education coordinator at your state education agency.*

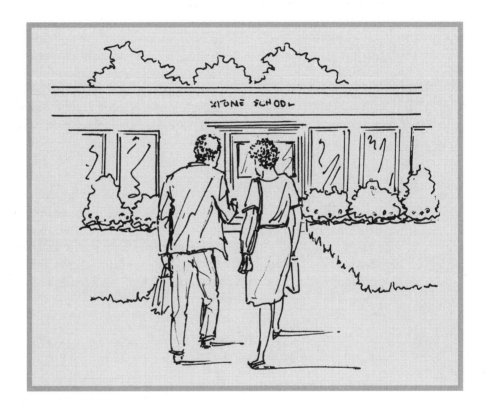

The authors also point out that few health curricula have undergone rigorous evaluation. They note that effective curricula share these common characteristics. These curricula:

- Are research based and theory driven.
- Incorporate basic, accurate information that is developmentally appropriate.
- Use interactive, experiential activities that actively engage students.
- Provide students with opportunities to model and practice relevant social skills.
- Address social or media influences on behaviors.
- Strengthen individual values and group norms that support health-enhancing behaviors.

- Are of sufficient duration to allow students to gain the needed knowledge and skills.
- Include teacher training that enhances effectiveness.

Please refer to the groundbreaking book *Health is Academic*, written by leading health educators, for guidance and courage as you proceed to develop and support a health program in your school for your teens. Please refer to Appendix 1 for an abbreviated version of an article about the payoffs for health education (see References and Resources section for an annotation of the article).

Health education can serve as an important web of influence between different segments of the community. For example, health-educated professionals can reach out to schools to serve on health committees and to teach students in their areas of expertise. This volunteering strengthens health education. The web is also supported by any citizen working with the teacher to present health education. Moreover, individuals in the community who believe in a comprehensive, well-balanced health curriculum for all students should volunteer to serve on local or district health committees. Schools find that providing accurate health materials related to lessons taught, broadly supports good health, and strengthens the web of health education even more securely. For a practical approach to the teaching of health education in secondary schools, please see Appendix 2, which details the efforts of one state in our nation.

Highly skilled citizens need to push for constructive strategies that benefit all children, in all academic areas, and especially in health-related education and services.

Family-School Partnerships

Researchers Evanthia N. Patrikakou and Roger P. Weissberg say educators must recognize that family-school partnerships are "integral to the process of learning and success of schooling." They maintain that teachers are the glue that holds the family-school partnership together.

While it may be true that "teachers are the glue," because every important endeavor needs leaders to set goals and work toward them, there is absolutely no reason why skillful parents and caregivers should not be the catalysts in the area of family-school collaboration. Highly skilled citizens at home, in business, and from health-related organzations need to push for constructive strategies that benefit all children, in all academic areas, and especially in health-related education and services.

Patrikakou and Weissberg have identified a "seven P" plan that helps us think about strategies and tools to enhance family-school involvement. These strategies are briefly outlined below, with comments:

1. Partnership as a priority. The mission statement of the school needs to state the importance of the family-school partnership. Teachers,

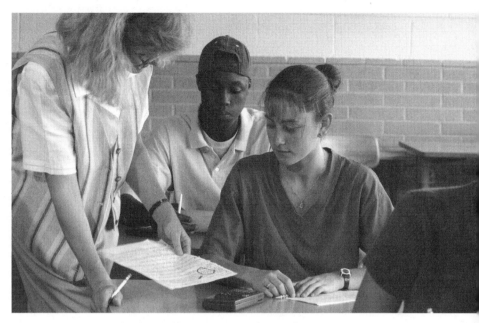

Dedicated teachers and parents provide "the glue" that builds family-school partnerships.

parents, and caregivers need training in how to facilitate family-school partnerships. Schools need to provide resources for this partnership to happen and need to recognize the current positive partnerships in place.

2. PLANNED EFFORT. Effective family-school partnerships are carefully planned and implemented. Taking time at the beginning of the school year to assess parents' needs, views, and patterns of school involvement is an essential first step.

3. PROACTIVE AND PERSISTENT COMMUNICATION. Schools need to find out the best way to communicate with parents, communicate regularly, and follow up. This means that every school should have its own specific plan for keeping connected to each parent or caregiver.

4. POSITIVE. The teacher needs to see your adolescent as a whole and to communicate positive news. Parents who receive good news from school have more opportunities to discuss successful experiences with their teens. And positive communication is often a two way street: Parents recognize and reinforce teacher efforts.

5. PERSONALIZED. Teachers should provide specific information about your adolescent's strengths and weaknesses, and also help you as a parent to understand these characteristics. This would be a helpful process, for example, whenever report cards are given out.

6. PRACTICAL SUGGESTIONS. The parent resource sheets that are an integral part of the *Michigan Model for Comprehensive School Health* are an excellent example of how teachers can provide practical, as well as life-saving, tips for parents of students who participate in health education classes.

7. PROGRAM MONITORING. Family-school partnerships need to be systematically evaluated in order for them to be improved and become more effective.

A large survey of parents in one state indicated that they wanted to receive health education at home in a four-page newsletter or in a two-page resource sheet. Another study showed parents willing to attend workshops with their adolescent, which would provide the opportunity to practice skills in the areas of communication, conflict resolution, and decision-making. In this study, over 80 percent of parents told the researchers that their high school had an important role to play in helping parents with teen problems. Hundreds of written remarks from parents and caregivers stressed the importance of good parent-school communication. The researchers heard about how much parents loved their children, and how they wanted teachers to care about their adolescents also.

Yet, another extensive evaluation of parent-school involvement in health education showed that school principals did not offer training to help parents learn to assist the teacher with health education classes, nor did they believe parents were interested. On the other hand, 80 percent of the parents responding said they would assist if asked, and over 20 percent were so eager, they provided the researchers with their names and telephone numbers. Schools need to take heed of research findings that show how much parents and caregivers want to invest time in their children's health education.

Public Agenda, a nonprofit, public opinion-based research group, released a parent-involvement-in-schools study that the group describes as being "as complex and subtle as any area we have examined." Most importantly, as Lois Jean White, current president of The National PTA (1999) says, "the survey reports that 74 percent of parents are more involved in their children's education than their own parents were."

White indicates that the Public Agenda research confirms a poll commissioned by The National PTA. She says, "Our study found that 91 percent of parents surveyed believe that it is extremely important for parents to be involved in their children's schools, and that 75 percent favor federal programs to help schools get parents more involved with their children's education."

Other polls have also indicated that parents have a great interest in school matters. Phi Delta Kappa, for example, conducted a poll with the Gallup Organization in 1998 and found that a majority of parents would like greater input in the allocation of school funds, the selection and hiring of administrators and principals, and the choice of curriculum offered.

White says the expanded online version of the Public Agenda poll points to the fact that a majority of parents feel comfortable evaluating the quality of their child's teachers, helping to decide budget issues, and participating in school management committees.

Here are some practical ideas for parents and caregivers to use as they work on family-school partnerships:

- Help to plan an upbeat, informative orientation for parents as their children enter either middle school or high school. A resource such as this book can be provided along with other helpful manuals that the school can distribute.

- Set up a resource center that contains the finest information you can locate about adolescent development, teen sexuality, communication skills, mental health, sexually-transmitted diseases, substance abuse, harassment, crime prevention and violence. Publish a descriptive list of these resources. Your school librarian, counselors, and psychologist can be invited to help on this project. References in this book give you a starting point. Be sure to stock lots of free pamphlets. You can also provide parenting classes and build a set of community resources where parents can find help. Ask for your principal's help from the very beginning and secure a space where parents feel welcome. You will be proud of your efforts.

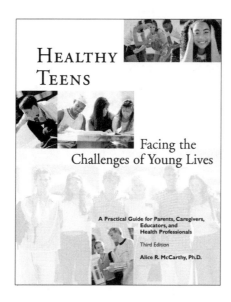

HEALTHY TEENS

Facing the Challenges of Young Lives

A Practical Guide for Parents, Caregivers, Educators, and Health Professionals

Third Edition

Alice R. McCarthy, Ph.D.

- Establish a training program for parents so they can really understand how curriculum is developed and chosen, why certain teaching methods are used; why students receive different levels of instruction and what tests young people take, when and why. Then ask for representation on various administrative decision-making committees.
- Remind adult family members that every activity, every club, every sport, needs sponsors and mentors who help to make opportunities for students worthwhile. You do not have to volunteer for drama, just because your ninth grader is in the school play—although you may want to! Parents can also introduce groups of students to their own hobby or life skill, and that includes volunteerism.

PARENT-TEACHER CONFERENCES

Many parents—and too many teachers—approach parent-teacher conferences with the kind of fear and dread usually reserved for root canals and IRS audits. Hopefully, the facts below will give you a fresh view and new optimism about parent-teacher conferences.

- Most teachers view parent-teacher conferences as a real chance to improve your teen's overall education and academic performance.
- Parent-teacher conferences are the single most important starting point for a working relationship between you, your teen's teacher, and your teen's school.
- Parent-teacher conferences are important at the high school level. More and more high schools are asking parents and other caring adults to attend conferences, and are scheduling conferences at times that are convenient for parents.

Getting Ready for Conferences

Talk with your teen before the conference. Put your teen at ease about the meeting by stressing that the conference is designed to make things better, not worse. You will want to discuss course work and homework, and ask if there is anything he or she would like you to discuss with the teacher.

Preparing for a parent-teacher conference serves two important functions. First, your questions, concerns, and hopes for your teen are all important to your teen's teacher. Second, being prepared can help put you at ease and help you and your teen's teacher set an effective agenda for the conference. Plan to be on time for the conference, and plan to end the conference on time. Plan to leave the conference with some specific next steps.

Before you go to the conference, jot down a few notes to yourself.

- Note anything about your family life, your teen, or your teen's

habits or outside interests that you think might be important for the teacher to know.
- Note any questions you might have about your teen's progress.
- Note any questions you might have about the school's programs or policies.
- Write down ideas about how you, your teen, and the teacher can work together to enhance your son or daughter's education.

Once You Are There

The questions below are adapted from an article written by Steven W. Enoch, a school system superintendent in California. The tips were originally written for teachers, but are presented here as questions for adults to ask of teachers. While this is not intended as a checklist, each question addresses a key point in your teen's educational development. Use them as a framework for your conference to provide a starting point for establishing an ongoing understanding with your teen's teacher.

- How are my teen's language skills developing in the areas of reading, writing, listening, and speaking? What can I do at home to help?

- In what areas is my teen making good academic progress? What areas need work?

- Can I see examples of my teen's work? (This can help illustrate and back up the teacher's feedback and evaluation.)

- Does my teen work well in group situations? Does my teen cooperate and interact well with others?

- Is my teen learning to think critically and creatively? In what ways?

- Can you give two or three specific goals to focus on that will help my teen develop academically?

- What kind of home practices will help my teen's academic work?

- Is there anything you need to know about my teen or my family in order to understand him or her better?

After the Conference

It is natural to judge your conference—on a scale of 1 to 10 or in simple words, like good, indifferent, or bad—and to want to reach some conclusions about your teen's school work as a result of the conference. You may even leave the conference angry or upset—feeling judged as a parent or caregiver—or feeling that the teacher did not see your teen in the right light. It is important not to spend too much time judging the conference or thinking about your feelings toward your teen's teacher. Instead, plan how to use the conference to help improve your teen's academic life.

Here are some tips to help you use a single conference—regardless of how you feel about its outcome—to help your teen and build a continuing relationship with your teen's teacher and school.

- What did I learn that I need to discuss with my teen?
- What home practices do I need to start or improve that will help my teen?
- Do I need to schedule a follow-up conference with the teacher to discuss any unresolved issues?
- Do I need to schedule an appointment with my teen's guidance counselor in order to act on any of the information I learned?

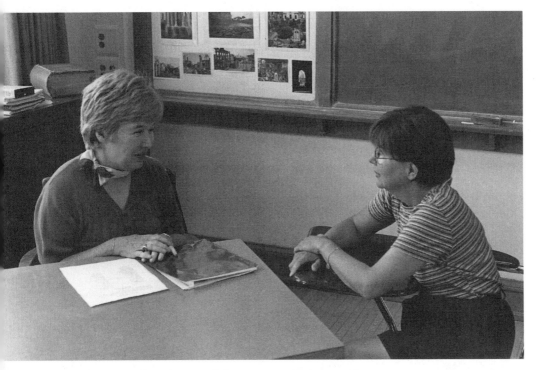

"What can I do at home to help my teen achieve more?"

SCHOOL COMMUNITY LINKAGES

The American Association of School Administrators published a booklet entitled *Preparing Schools and School Systems for the 21st Century: Council of 21* in 1999 that outlines school-community linkages. The report notes: "How effectively schools educate students has a profound impact on a community's future. How well a community supports its schools will determine, in a large measure, how effective they can be. In short, schools and school systems, are . . . linked to communities they serve and vice versa." The chapter entitled *School-Community Linkages* outlines the following characteristics for schools of the 21st century:

- Parents are engaged in the learning process—for their children's education as well as their own.
- Schools are "around-the-clock" hubs for lifelong learning that enhance education and achievements for everyone in the community.
- Investing in education is supported by all corporate and community leaders.
- Teachers and parents work together to increase student performance.
- Schools are linked to healthcare, housing, social services, and other community agencies.
- Parents clearly understand their responsibilities.
- Learning experiences occur within a framework of real-life issues and challenges.
- Students are engaged in community service, service learning, and work experience.
- Educators bring expertise and resources from the community into the schools.
- Schools are connected electronically with the world at large and serve as community learning centers.

There is no way that all these linkages can occur without the extensive involvement of people from outside the schools. The serious commitment of parents, caregivers, and health professionals from the community, plus many community institutions that offer health services and information, can provide a model of involvement in school health education. This model will set the pace for citizens and community involvement in other academic spheres. Therein lies the challenge for both the community and the school. Each must assume new responsibilities to ensure the success of future citizens of the 21st century.

REFERENCES AND RESOURCES   R/R

Beyond the Classroom: Why School Reform Has Failed, What Parents Need to Do, Laurence Steinberg
(Touchstone Books, 1997, $12.00). Observing that 15 years of school reform hadn't produced
improvement in U.S. students' test scores, Steinberg and associates decided to examine other
aspects of youngsters' lives. For three school years, 1987-90, they tracked kids in nine public high
schools representative of middle America's ethnic and economic profiles. They report that, to
reverse the dumbing of America, parents, peers, and cultural attitudes now need to change more
than schools do. Too many parents ignore their children's education—and then so do the children.
Without "authoritative" parenting (described herein) and definite scholastic standards, children tend
to socialize too much with peer groups, most of which encourage just getting by in school.

Breaking Ranks: Changing an American Institution, National Association of Secondary School Principals (1904
Association Drive, Reston, VA 22091-1537; 800-253-7746, 1996, $19.50.
The report of the Association in partnership with the Carnegie Foundation for the Advancement
of Teaching on the high school of the 21st century.

Caring Communities Network. A school-linked/school-based process whereby integrated systems are
designed through families, schools and local citizens. Web site: www.modmh.state.mo.us/
homeinfo/progs/caring/better.html.

Great Transitions: Preparing Adolescents for a New Century, Carnegie Council on Adolescent Development
(Carnegie Corp, 1995, $6.00). Available online at Web site: www.carnegie.org/reports/great_
transitions/gr_exec.html.

Health Is Academic: A Guide to Coordinated School Health Programs, ed. Eva Marx and Susan Frelick Wooley with
Daphne Northrop (Teacher's College Press, 1998, $24.95). The book, which provides state-of-the art
information related to developing health education in schools, successfully makes the case that
our children's health status and their ability to learn are inextricably linked. It argues that
coordinated school health programs are a vehicle by which the educational promise of all America's
children can be realized.

*How to Help Your Child with Homework: Every Caring Parent's Guide to Encouraging Good Study Habits and Ending
the Homework Wars*, Marguerite C. Radencich and Jeanne Shay Schumm (Free Spirit Publishing, 1997,
$14.95). This award-winning book offers parents and caregivers proven strategies and techniques
to help their children (ages 6-13) succeed in school, while making homework more bearable, if
not downright pleasant. For parents who feel their own academic skills are rusty, the book offers
a practical "how to" with subject-by-subject explanations on everything from math and spelling to
foreign languages and formal assignments.

Infobrief: An Information Brief of the Association for Supervision and Curriculum Development (ASCD) Issue 17,
May 1999. A 1999 statement from the ASCD that supports a coordinated health education program.
Thoughtful and helpful summary of some of the issues facing schools as they seek to fund and
integrate health fully into education.

Innovations in Parent and Family Involvement, J. William Rioux and Nancy Berla (Eye on Education Inc., 1993,
$39.95). Leading advocates of parent involvement write a definitive book. Chapter five gives
examples of successful programs in high schools. Strategies and tips for those who want their
program to work.

*Keeping Schools Open As Community Learning Centers: Extending Learning in a Safe, Drug-Free Environment Before
and After School.* (Partnership for Family Involvement in Education, National Community Education
Association, U.S. Dept of Education, 1999; 800-USA-LEARN, Web site: www.ed.gov). This outstanding new guidebook focuses on the importance of keeping schools open as after-school and summer
community learning centers. Parents can read this free booklet and be inspired and challenged by
the examples and practical solutions to barriers they may encounter; principals and other stake
holders in children's education will find the material explicit and directive. Excellent listing of

community organizations to involve, and help from the federal government. Any well-organized group of parents, with school and community leaders, could initiate a learning center for their school using this free booklet.

A Load Off Teachers' Backs: Coordinated School Health Programs, Harriet Tyson (Kappan Special Report, January 1999, Web site: www.pdkintl.org/kappan, purchase 50 copies for $15.00 or 100 copies for $25.00, 800-766-1156, or write Special Report Reprints, *Phi Delta Kappan,* PO Box 789, Bloomington IN 47402). This full and thoughtful report makes a compelling connection between poor physical and mental health conditions in students, and lack of academic success. Brilliant in its persuasiveness, the article pushes hard for a coordinated school health program and its payoff. See excerpt from this article in Appendix I of this book. Developed under contract with Education Development Center, Inc., Newton, Massachusetts.

Matter of Time: Risk and Opportunity in the Out-of-School Hours, (Carnegie Council on Adolescent Development, Carnegie Corporation of New York, 1992, $13.00). A partnership needs to look at school use after formal school hours. An extraordinary booklet.

NASSP Bulletin, November 1998, Vol. 82 No. 601 (National Association of Secondary School Principals, 1904 Association Drive, Reston, VA, 20191-1537, 703-860-0200). The November 1998 *Bulletin* is devoted to school health issues. As Eugenia C. Potter, editor, states, "...the *NASSP Bulletin* hopes this month's theme on School Heath Issues will help make both middle level and high schools better, safer, and healthier places for their students."

National Middle School Association, (2600 Corporate Exchange Drive, Columbus OH 43231-1672, 800-528-NMSA). Free catalogue filled with books for parents, teachers, administrators, and counselors covering a wide range of topics, including instructional planning, curriculum revision, teacher education, and family and community issues. Also available are the *Middle School Journal,* which reports on current research, trends, and professional ideas for middle school educators, and *High Strides,* which is a national publication for the urban middle school.

The New American Family and the School, J. Howard Johnston (National Middle School Association, 4807 Evanswood Dr., Columbus, OH 43229, 1990, $6.00). Frank, to-the-point. Be sure to read the chapter on barriers to home-school cooperation.

New Approaches to the Organization of Health and Social Services in Schools, J.D. Dryfoos. Appendix D in *Institute of Medicine Schools and Health: Our Nation's Investment,* pp. 365-415 (National Academy Press, 1997). Already a classic in the health education field. Especially for those who want students to have health clinics and other services in or near schools.

Partnership for Family Involvement in Education. (Education Publications Center, U.S. Dept of Education, PO Box 1398, Jessup, MD 20794-1398; 877-433-7827, 877-576-7734 (TTY/TDD), 301-470-1244 (fax), E-mail address: edpubs@inet.ed.gov. Web site: www.ed.gov/pubs/edpubs.html). Free packet of excellent thinking material to help parents, caregivers, and schools move forward in partnership.

Preparing Schools and School Systems for the 21st Century: Council of 21, John Glenn, Honorary Chair, (American Association of School Administrators, 1999, Web site: www.aasa.org). Here is a blueprint with 12 excellent easy-to-digest chapters that can be used by administrators and parent leaders to help work out a plan for preparing students for the "global knowledge/information age." This is a useful and important document. Parents take heed.

Promising Initiatives to Improve Education in Your Community: A Minicatalog of U.S. Department of Education Programs and Free Publications, U.S. Department of Education, 1999. ED Pubs, Education Publications Center, U.S. Department of Education, PO Box 1398, Jessup MD 20794-1398. 877-4ED-Pubs (English/Spanish), 877-576-7734 (TDD), or 800-437-0833. 301-470-1244 (fax). The purpose of this minicatalog is to provide you with resources to build partnerships that improve education in your community. It lists publications, with annotation, from ED Pubs/U.S. Dept of Education, including videos, kits, brochures, and posters. It also contains a wealth of additional sources of information: Web sites, Department-funded clearinghouses, and organizations. E-mail address: edpubs@inet.ed.gov. Web site: www.ed.gov/ pubs/edpubs.html.

Reducing the Risk: Connections That Make a Difference in the Lives of Youth, Robert Wm. Blum and Peggy Mann
Rinehart, 1997. For a copy, contact: Reducing the Risk, Adolescent Health Program, University of
Minnesota, Box 721 UMHC, 420 Delaware Street SE, Minneapolis MN 55445 or e-mail to:
ahp@maroon.tc.umn.edu. Document is based on the first analysis of Add Health data from the
National Longitudinal Study of Adolescent Health. Add Health Web site: www.cpc.unc.edu/addhealth.

The Scapegoat Generation: America's War on Adolescents, Mike A. Males (Common Courage Press, P.O. Box 702,
Monroe, Maine 04951, 1996, $17.95). A must-read for anyone interested in redefining both modern
adolescence and the challenge faced by all Americans to ensure the next generation's future.

School and Family Partnerships: Preparing Educators and Improving Schools, Joyce L. Epstein (Harpercollins, 1999,
$25.00). How can teachers and administrators prepare themselves to create positive relationships
and productive partnerships with families? The work of Joyce Epstein has helped to advance parent
involvement in schooling. Here she offers educators a framework for building comprehensive
programs for school and family partnerships.

School, Family, and Community Partnerships: Your Handbook for Action, Joyce L. Epstein, ed. (Corwin Press, 1997,
$29.95). This book guides all schools in designing a positive, permanent partnership program that
will help everyone focus on student learning and school success. Based on many years of research
and over 12 years of field-testing, this handbook guides you through the process of planning,
implementing, and maintaining a successful partnership between your school, students, families, and
the community.

The Seven P's of School-Family Partnerships, Evanthia N. Patrikakou and Roger P. Weissberg (Education Week,
Feb. 3, 1999, pp 34-36). The school-family partnerships project at the University of Illinois at Chicago,
a collaborative site of the Mid-Atlantic Regional Laboratory for Student Success at Temple University
in Philadelphia, has been developing strategies and materials for teachers in an effort to cut down
on time constraints and increase the awareness of issues involved in parent-teacher relationships.
This is a "must read" for administrators, teachers and parents that affirms the importance of the
family-school partnership as an integral part of children's success in school.

Strong Families, Strong Schools: Building Community Partnerships for Learning (U.S. Dept of Education, 600
Independence Ave SW, Washington, DC 20202, 800-USA-LEARN for free copy). Be sure to send
for this 50-page, well-designed booklet with the most important message you could read: "How
important families and communities are to the success of our children in school."

Teaching the New Basic Skills: Principles for Educating Children to Thrive in a Changing Economy, Richard J. Murane
and Frank Levy (Free Press, 1996, $24.00). Drawing on the work of real teachers, parents, and
administrators, this book provides a blueprint for turning our schools around.

The Teen Trip: The Complete Resource Guide, Gayle Kimball and over 1500 young people (Equality Press, 1997,
$16.95). This is a comprehensive resource, with young people reporting their experiences related to
the many issues that contemporary teens experience. Dr. Kimball adds information, telephone help
lines, organizations, internet resources, and references. Note: Parents and caregivers should read
this book before giving to their teen; the young writers are very frank.

The 10th School: Where School-Family-Community Partnerships Flourish, Don Davies (Education Week, July 10,
1996). Exactly what can be done to make your school the one out of 10 in which collaboration
between teachers and administrators and families and communities is commonplace. Worth a trip
to the library, or ask your principal for a copy.

This We Believe, (National Middle School Association 800-528-NMSA, order #0202, $6.00). Outlines how to
create good middle schools.

What Americans Believe Students Should Know: A Survey of U.S. Adults, R.J. Marzano, J.S. Kendall, L.F. Cicchinelli
(www.mcrel.org/survey, 1998).

Chapter 3
Teens and Mental Health

This chapter focuses on the psychological development that takes place during adolescence as your child learns how to reason, form opinions and make decisions. It also focuses on the symptoms of some of the mental disorders that may become apparent during the teen years, such as depression and bipolar disorder, how to prevent teen suicide, and what to do about eating disorders and learning disabilities.

Psychological Health and the Development of Your Teen

Starting at age 11 or 12, your young adolescent begins to reason and to develop emotionally. Don't expect that ability to advance smoothly. It takes time, for example, for young people to get better at logical thinking and reasoning as they advance through middle and late adolescence. Try to keep in mind that now you have a person in your home who is taking new and advanced classes in school. Advancing ability can mean challenging your thinking, and pointing out flaws in your judgement. You may get drawn into debates about issues that you had long ago decided upon. Think of this questioning period as one of intellectual, emotional, and social development. Try to encourage thinking and emotional maturity.

Stop worrying about losing control. Think about drawing on your own problem-solving skills and model these for your teen. In some health classes, problem solving and decision making are taught as early as third grade. Try to place emphasis on developing these skills. The lively debate sessions you may be having bring into play not just consideration of what is a good or bad decision, but may be based on moral values and abstract thinking. Your child begins to reason about the lives of others, the fate of people across the nation and the world. It takes two to quarrel. You can probably control your responses and your temper more easily than your adolescent can.

You can be respectful of the arguments put forth by your young, middle or late adolescent. Arguments are often not about the issues on the table, but whether or not you believe your adolescent is mature enough to do what he or she wants to do, and accept the consequences. It is really a test of whether you trust your son's or daughter's decision-making skills.

> Arguments are often not about the issues on the table, but whether or not you believe your adolescent is mature enough to do what he or she wants to do.

Parent/child disagreements seem to increase in early adolescence. It is at this time, especially, that parents may receive criticism—accompanied by silence and secrecy. While this behavior is normal and will probably be short lived, keep in mind that running away, joining a gang, drug abuse, and skipping school is not normal behavior at any time in adolescence.

What to Expect

Experts in adolescent behavior say that your adolescent wants to control who she or he is as well as what she or he does. And that includes what she or he thinks. They say you can expect some or all of the following:

REJECTION: Be prepared for your son or daughter to reject your efforts to be loving (especially in public), kind, and considerate. These efforts remind adolescents of when they were little folk and now they are big folk!

NOT WANTING TO BE SEEN WITH YOU: Just try to be tolerant of this. Again, this is an issue of wanting to be independent and grown up.

CLOSED DOORS: Do not pry. The way adolescents mature is to keep their thoughts to themselves. Eventually you'll hear plenty about what they believe. Keep in mind, however, that clearly monitoring teens' internet use, chat room activity, video game usage, and television viewing, continues to be the responsibility of the parent/caregiver.

FRIENDS ARE MORE IMPORTANT THAN YOU: Think of the friends of teens as helping them have new experiences, and reaching out into a different world than your family. The same goes for their attachment to your best friend or a relative. The experience of different people expands thinking and develops understanding of others. This is positive mental health development.

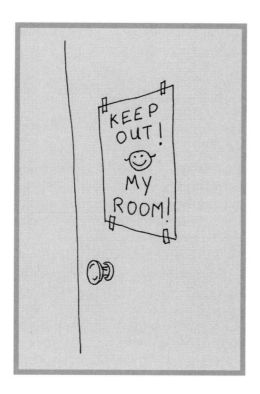

TESTS OF AUTHORITY: If you accept that your teen needs more and more independence while moving along the path from early adolescence to late adolescence, you'll have an easier time. Teens do want to know how you think and feel, but they want to become independent of you. You want that too. Don't be hurt or upset by your adolescent seeking independence. Keep in mind that you are moving through a stage with your adolescents when you can't solve all their problems, or keep them from making foolish mistakes. What you can do is to say "no" when you are certain the mistake will cause serious difficulties, harm, or injury.

While your adolescent may give you a hard time, they appreciate limits. They want to be able to say, "my step-father would kill me if he thought I got a girl pregnant (or if I drank alcohol)." The recent National Longitudinal Study of Adolescent Health (Add Health Study) of 90,000 youngsters has shown that without a doubt, kids want you to set limits. For example, Dr. James Jaccard, one of the lead researchers, said: "Children are much less likely to engage in sexually risky behavior if their parents talk about a broad set of reasons for not doing so." It is pretty simple: limit setting by an adult shows your teen you care. It teaches your adolescent self-control, which is a foundation for keeping on an even keel and becoming mentally healthy. Please try not to cut off conversation by getting in that "I always know best" mode. Talking, even heated arguments—about sex and drugs—help your teen to get their values and beliefs out in the open. And they are taking in your family values even if it doesn't seem that way. A mentally healthy adult helps their teen to become grounded in a strong sense of self and the ability to make wise decisions.

STRESS AND THE HEALTH OF YOUR ADOLESCENT

The adult world is full of situations and events that cause stress—company downsizing, marital tension and divorce, the death of a parent or child, serious illness or injury, and unexpected bills.

For your teen, stressful events might include parents' divorce, abuse or neglect, poverty, school failure, illness, or changes and losses in relationships. Even positive events can create a degree of stress—such as moving to a new home or school, or beginning a job. Life today presents some families with more stress than we want or need. The age of the computer, marked by instant information and images, seems to increase expectations that we can accomplish more, rather than making life easier, as we always thought it would.

While your adolescent may give you a hard time, they appreciate limits.

The ability to evaluate stress levels and to develop coping skills increases for teens as they grow older and wiser. It's not the situation that causes all the stress. Our beliefs about the situation are a big piece of the puzzle.

It is important to distinguish daily life hurdles from significant stress. Parents and teens experience such common difficulties as waiting in line, changes in daily routine, rescheduling appointments, and conflicts with family members or friends. Teens usually learn strategies to effectively cope with these small hassles. Significant stressors, such as the death of a friend or a serious illness, are more likely to catch your adolescent unable to cope. These events can result in serious consequences for physical and emotional well-being.

While life's ordinary hurdles generally have less negative consequences, the cumulative effect of many such difficulties can be as detrimental as any single traumatic event. The perception of stress is also related to experience and development—what is stressful for one person may not even amount to a small difficulty for another.

Stress in both early and middle teenagers is usually caused by:

- New, unfamiliar, or unpredictable situations—moving from middle school to high school.
- Unclear expectations—teachers who give vague assignments.
- Expectations of something unpleasant—what will happen when my best friend finds out I lost his or her jacket.
- Fear of failure—not making the honor roll; failing algebra.
- Major developmental "hurdles"—not understanding how the body develops in puberty.

- Teasing and bullying—the character of teasing can change over time and by middle school and high school may become hostile and hurtful. When done deliberately to provoke or humiliate, teasing becomes bullying. Victims of chronic teasing and bullying are more likely to have poor grades, and not want to attend school. Some students become anxious and depressed, and a small minority may have thoughts of suicide or of killing their tormentors.

Symptoms of Stress in Teens

Your teen's response to stress may include more attention-seeking behaviors, mood changes, avoidance of certain activities, isolation (such as the adolescent who retreats more and more to his or her room), refusing to go to school or failure to prepare for class, sleeping difficulties, and physical complaints (headache, stomach ache).

What can Parents or Caregivers Do?

DO NOT PLACE UNDUE EXPECTATIONS ON YOUR TEEN. We all want our teens to be successful, and we should have expectations for their behavior and performance. But when stress starts to show itself, it may be time to question if our expectations are too high.

LISTEN TO YOUR ADOLESCENT WHEN HE OR SHE DESCRIBES EVENTS OR SITUATIONS. Being a good listener will, first of all, reassure your son or daughter that you are there with love and support. Moreover, it will help you to better understand how you can help. What may seem a trivial issue to you is not trivial to your teen.

TEACH YOUR CHILD GOOD PROBLEM-SOLVING SKILLS. The feeling that we have too much to do in the amount of time available to us is a frequent cause of stress. When overburdened, we have difficulty seeing how to get ourselves out of the jam we're in. Help your teen learn to break big problems into smaller ones that can be dealt with one at a time. Talk about how you have handled stressful situations. Students in health education classes learn early about problem-solving skills and practice these skills. Inquire at your school about what your middle school and high school student is learning in health education about problem-solving and decision-making skills, and reinforce that learning. Practice problem-solving with your adolescent.

REHEARSE STRESSFUL SITUATIONS. If speaking in front of a class or making a phone call to an adult is a cause for stress, it can be helpful to talk through the event with your child. Discuss how he or she wants the event to take place, and then go through the situation together in a "trial run." Possible difficulties can be "problem-solved" together.

BE AWARE OF "IRRATIONAL THINKING" PATTERNS. Sometimes we can overhear our teens "thinking aloud" with sentences like "If I don't do this extra assignment, I'll never get into college." More frequently, only the first part of the sentence is there: "I have to do what the other kids are doing," "I shouldn't really be reading this novel just for fun right now," or "I need to get this whole list of things finished right now." Often hidden behind such thoughts are unfounded beliefs such as "If I don't live up to my teacher's expectations, I'll never be a success in life," or "If friends get mad at me, then that confirms that I'm not a good person." Deep down, these "if ... then" statements frequently hide core beliefs that young people accept as true, even if they have never questioned them logically. These are beliefs like "I'm not a very loveable person," or "The world is a cruel place, and the only way to survive is by doing everything perfectly." If you become aware of harmful beliefs, help your adolescent to look at life events more realistically and more positively.

Teach tools to deal with teasing and bullying, as follows:

- INSTILL PRIDE. Help your adolescent develop positive self-esteem by talking about, and encouraging pride in, his or her unique abilities, skills, and qualities. These abilities may be in academics, in sports, or in developing a "niche of expertise" such as a debate, drama, playing a musical instrument, leading a scout troop, or volunteering in your religious community.

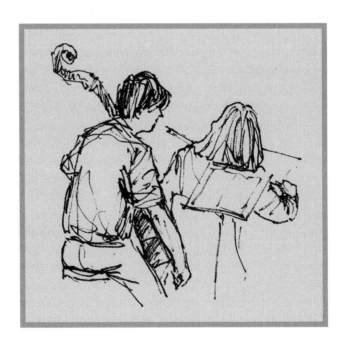

- TEACH YOUR TEEN TO LISTEN TO THE TONE, NOT THE WORDS. The teaser's tone of voice is a good indicator of motive. When teasing is meant to be funny, your adolescent can try to laugh along, take the teasing in stride, and offer appropriate rejoinders. That is because when he or she shows hurt feelings, the teaser often perceives this as a weakness and may continue to harass more relentlessly. Hostile-sounding voices, however, suggest the teaser's motives are mean-spirited. When encountering such situations, your young person should be taught to tell the instigators to "stop it," to walk away, or to seek help from an adult.

- TEACH ASSERTIVENESS, NOT AGGRESSIVENESS. Some parents and caregivers think it is best for their child to confront the bully, but there is a difference between being assertive and being aggressive. A passive response such as appearing hurt or upset can set the stage for later confrontations. A "duke it out" reaction rarely solves the problem and may result in bloodshed and school suspensions. Moreover, there is no guarantee that the harassment will stop; it may even escalate. A better approach is to teach firm but nonviolent responses, such as "I don't like the way you are treating me."

- MODEL APPROPRIATE BEHAVIOR. Unexplained injuries, torn clothing, or claims of "lost" belongings should make you suspicious. Please inquire and follow up with authorities at school.

- TEENS WHO WITNESS ADULTS HANDLING CONFLICT APPROPRIATELY AND SUCCESSFULLY ARE MORE LIKELY TO COPY THIS BEHAVIOR. Conflict resolution skills are taught in health education; make inquiry about this teaching with your principal. Your school personnel need to be notified of hostile teasing and bullying. Be assured these professionals do not want this type of harassment happening to your teen.

- CLIQUES CAN HAVE A DEVASTATING EFFECT ON A YOUNG PERSON'S SENSE OF WELL-BEING IN MIDDLE, JUNIOR, OR HIGH SCHOOL. Teens in cliques that exclude other teens can become bullies. Please work carefully with school personnel on this issue on behalf of all teens. Be sure each young person is accepted.

TEACH RELAXATION TECHNIQUES. There are a number of relaxation tapes on the market. All of them emphasize the importance of sitting or lying down and breathing slowly from deep in the stomach. A frequently-used visualization technique is that of relaxing, and then imagining oneself in a favorite place—a place that is warm and inviting, comfortable and beautiful. Relaxation can be especially effective when used in conjunction with the rehearsal of a stressful situation before it occurs. Ideas to discuss with your teen are found in the accompanying box.

Seeking Help

Don't be embarrassed to seek help for your teen if you observe stress symptoms that do not go away. Your family physician, local health department, school clinic, school psychologist, social worker, or school counselor are good places to find resources for help.

Managing Stress

- Sit back and count to ten.

- Take a walk, jog, or exercise.

- Use positive "self talk"—"I disagree, but I can cool down and talk to her."

- Write down why you are angry, upset, or sad. Think through a plan and write the plan down.

- Talk to someone about your feelings.

- Listen to quiet music.

- Inhale a deep breath through your nose and hold for five seconds. Slowly exhale through your mouth as if blowing out a candle. Repeat several times.

DEPRESSIVE ILLNESSES

Depression affects over 1.5 million adult Americans each year, yet only about one-third of those affected get treatment. Ironically, among all psychiatric illnesses—which is what depression is—depression is among the most responsive to treatment. Given the huge rise in teen suicide rates over the last 25 years, families need to know about depressive illnesses just as they know about other illnesses and health factors that affect teens. While depression has a genetic component, it is often triggered by situations and stresses that people perceive as hopeless.

Serious depression, usually called clinical depression, is not something for adults or teens to treat alone. At the very least, teens don't have the time to stop their lives, to suffer at home, to miss school, and to endure the whole-body pain that comes with depression. At the worst, untreated depression can lead to suicide.

Recognizing Depression

Sorting out the signs of depression, as opposed to the normal mood swings of adolescence, is hard. Often times, adults see the signs of depression as a phase their teen is going through. Some people mistakenly believe that dealing with depression is a matter of will, something a person could "snap out of" if they "just wanted to." Alcohol and drug abuse greatly complicate matters.

Many teens see depression as a weakness and therefore something to hide. Most teens will have trouble, especially if they are depressed, connecting their emotional state to their behavior. That helps explain why poor school performance is often the first indicator of a more serious problem. In general, teens are better at saying how they feel, while adults are better observers of their teen's behavior.

Signs of Depression

Seek professional help for your teen if you notice five or more of the following symptoms for two weeks or longer.

- A change in school performance.
- Inability to concentrate.
- Irritability or anger.
- Persistent unhappiness.
- Change in eating and sleeping habits.
- Withdrawal from people and activities.
- Excessive guilt or anxiety.
- Physical complaints.
- Aggressive, impulsive, or risk-taking behavior.
- Thoughts or talk of death or suicide.

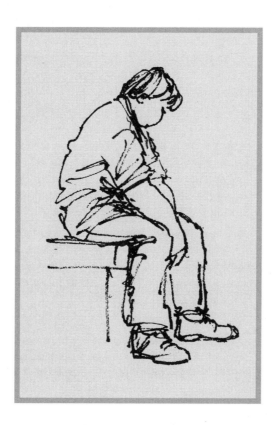

Bipolar Disorder

Bipolar disorder (formerly called manic-depression) is the most severe form of depression, and usually begins in adolescence or early adulthood. One way to think about this illness is in terms of a cycle or wave of moods. At the bottom of the wave is depression. The middle of the wave is normal. Higher up, there is mild mania, a time of more energy, ideas, and sometimes more sex drive. At the crest of the wave is mania, a period marked by rocketing energy, overflowing thoughts and emotions, and often serious behavior problems and periods of marked poor judgement. In adolescence, parents and caregivers need to be aware that the manic phase consists more commonly of periods of irritability. The adolescent has rage attacks, extreme mood swings, and commits violent acts.

For many people suffering from bipolar disorder, life is a roller coaster that either won't start or starts going too fast, with normal periods sandwiched between. Luckily, there are many effective treatments for bipolar disorder.

Complicating Factors

As with depression, the family's greatest barrier in getting an accurate diagnosis of bipolar disorder may be denial that there is a problem. Adding to that may be alcohol and/or drug use by the teen.

> Sorting out the signs of depression, as opposed to the normal mood swings of adolescence, is hard.

Adults with mental health issues are 2.7 times more likely to have an alcohol or other substance abuse problem than are other people in the population. Adults with alcohol or drug problems are 4.5 times more likely to have some sort of underlying mental health problem. To complicate matters just a little more, "self-medication" with alcohol and drugs is fairly typical of people with bipolar disorder.

Drugs like cocaine are often used as a means to fight depression: alcohol is often used to fight periods of mania or as short-term relief against depression. Self-medication not only doesn't work, it actually hides the symptoms of depression or bipolar disorder, and can make effective treatment of either illness almost impossible.

Any treatment for depression or bipolar disorder needs to include a close look at any alcohol or drug use. Alcohol and drug use—especially if used while taking medication for either illness—complicates an already difficult medical problem and throws a monkey wrench into any medical or therapeutic solution to the problem. If your teen is experiencing problems with depression, he or she needs you to get very serious about any alcohol or drug use.

Causes of Depression

Depression can result from many factors. The critical issue is how your adolescent feels the family is functioning and how supported he or she feels.

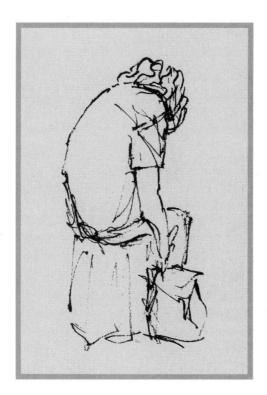

Factors that can influence depression in your young person include poverty, victimization, family dysfunction, and the expectations society holds for young people. Poverty forces parents into a survival struggle, full of stress and frustration. It's hard to provide extra support and involvement in your teen's life when you are scrambling to put food on the table and buy shoes.

Assault, rape, and other crimes against teens have been associated with depression. Teens, for example, who have been sexually abused, are more likely to suffer from depression and other emotional disorders, or to run away from home.

Parents and caregivers hoping to enhance the ability of teens for what they perceive as a fast-paced world of cyberspace and economic growth may push their young people too hard. This stress can be a factor in creating depression in your adolescent.

It appears almost impossible to pinpoint the critical causing factor in teen depression: family genetics or what their environment provides. Research suggests that families can transmit depressive disorders to their children through genes. Sometimes, depression is caused by an imbalance in the chemicals in the brain. Environmental factors count too—if families find it impossible to love and care for their adolescent, or if there is constant difficulty between partners or among family members, or if there is a divorce, depression may result. Good friends and acceptance by peers appears to help adolescents of all ages ward off depression.

Treatment of Depression

Early and accurate diagnosis of depressive illnesses is important because depression can lead to school failure or to suicide.

Depression must be distinguished from normal sadness, adjustment disorders, learning disabilities, anxiety deficit disorder, and all the factors that may be present in your adolescent's life. A physical examination may be needed to rule out the possibility of an infection, hormonal problems, or gastrointestinal problems.

If the depression has a biological basis, antidepressant medications may be helpful. The delay in the use of medication has resulted in the waste of teen lives. Too often medications are seen as a last resort. One wouldn't hold such a view if the illness were diabetes or high blood pressure.

Besides medication, many types of psychotherapy can be used to treat depression. Supportive therapy offers reassurance, empathy, and advice to parents and adolescents. Cognitive therapists try to change the adolescent's pessimistic attitudes and disheartening automatic thoughts by challenging the justifications for them. Interpersonal therapy takes account of the teenager's need to identify and resolve personal disputes arising at a time of life when important choices have to be made.

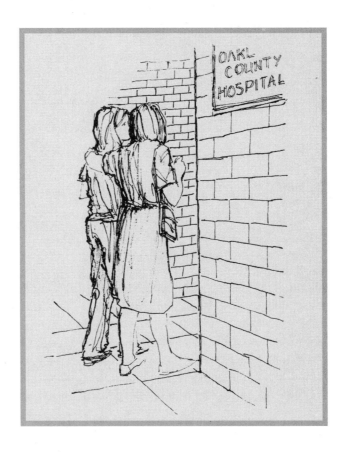

Therapists who work with depressed adolescents usually also see the parents and caregivers. Families can be educated about depression and especially its hereditary background. They can learn how to respond without making the symptoms worse and how to solve problems created by depression.

- In any instance where you think your teen may be suffering from depression, seek a psychiatrist or psychologist who is experienced in working with depressed adolescents.
- Seek professional help immediately, regardless of whether or not you think your teen is depressed, if your teen talks about wanting to die or wishing that he or she were dead.

What your School Can Do

The award-winning *Michigan Model for Comprehensive School Health Education* places emphasis on stress reduction, coping, problem-solving, substance abuse and violence prevention, and safety, along with physical health (see Appendix 2). In addition, you may want to work with your school to develop specific lessons for students that explain depressive illness. This can help your adolescent understand this disorder and help prevent more serious illness and suicide. Parents and caregivers can work with school leaders to encourage health education for all teens. They can also assist in developing parenting sessions to help adults understand depression.

Suicide

It's probably one of the most terrifying thoughts a parent or caregiver can have about their teen: suicide. No one wants to think that their teen would take his or her life, but estimates show that teen suicide has tripled since 1995 with as many as 2,500 teens committing suicide yearly. Suicide is the third leading cause of death for young people between the ages of 15 and 24.

Talking about suicide does not increase its possibility. Helping your adolescent understand the warning signals of suicide may save the life of a friend of your teen.

Teens are in a transitional period between childhood and adulthood, and this can lead to confusion and anxiety at times. Teens with an adequate support network of friends, family, religious affiliation, peer groups, or extra-curricular activities may have a sufficient outlet to deal with their everyday frustrations. Teens without an adequate support network, however, may feel disconnected and isolated from their family and peer group. It's these teens who are at risk for suicide if they are unable to deal with their problems.

Doctors at the American Psychiatric Association (APA) say that teens considering suicide often face problems that are out of their control—divorce, alcoholism of a family member, or exposure to domestic violence, for example. A family history of depression or suicide is a significant risk factor. Since depressive illnesses may have a genetic component, some teens may be predisposed to suffer major depression. Feelings of helplessness and worthlessness may accompany the depression.

Please read this section carefully. In doing so you can learn the warning signs about suicide, be prepared to talk more openly about suicide with your teen, and answer your adolescent's questions. Talking about suicide does not increase its possibility. Helping your adolescent understand the warning signals of suicide may save the life of a friend of your teen.

Situations that Can Make Teens Feel Hopeless

As might be expected, family problems are significant factors in youth suicide. These problems include longstanding stress from poverty, physical and mental abuse, drug and alcohol abuse in the family, divorce, and other legal problems.

Family issues that are preceptors to a suicide attempt include the death of a much-loved family member, such as a grandparent, or serious conflict with brothers and sisters. A teen may be in despair about an illness or injury. Depression can be a major factor but is not always the deciding one in suicide.

Difficulties with gender or sexual identity issues can be overwhelming to adolescents. Lack of information about such issues, societal intolerance, a sense of alienation/isolation from peers, peer pressure or harassment, and internalized disdain are all potential contributing factors to depression or suicide attempts for youth who are questioning their sexual identity. Gay and lesbian youth are two to three times more likely to attempt suicide than heterosexual young people. Up to 30 percent of teen suicides may have to do with sexual identity issues.

Events, sometimes school-related, can push an adolescent to think about suicide. There may be endless clashes with parents about grades, troubles with teachers, failing grades, or failure to make the cut off for joining a team.

A perceived or real public humiliation, failure to achieve an expected goal, or any kind of loss such as loss of a job or of a relationship—things adults may see as troublesome or even trivial in the lives of their teen—are often extremely traumatic in the life of your adolescent. Communication with that teen is critical to help the teen feel that they can survive the situation.

Some teens never make a single suicide attempt, but live their lives in chronic alienation from their family and society. They constantly pursue high-risk behaviors such as alcohol and drug abuse, unprotected sex, and driving drunk without a seat belt.

Researchers have identified seven motives for suicide attempts among adolescents:

- A cry for help to get assistance related to the kinds of family or other problems they feel incapable of solving—the most common motive.
- Making amends for having done something they think is unpardonable.
- Rejoining a lost loved one, whether a person or pet they were close to or an idolized person they didn't even know, like a rock star.

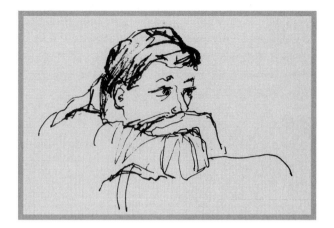

- A kind of blackmail to get better treatment. For example, the thinking may be "If I threaten to hurt myself, they'll be nice to me."
- Getting back for real or imagined abandonment, either physical or emotional.
- An intense rage at others that is directed at the self.
- Mental illness or personality disorganization.

When Should I Be Concerned?

Most teens that attempt suicide give either obvious or subtle warning signs that they are about to do so. While it may be upsetting to think of talking about suicidal thoughts with your youngster, that conversation is also a ray of hope.

It is important to listen—really listen—take your time and let your teen talk. Don't argue, act judgmental or preach. Stay right with your young person—especially if you believe he or she is in danger of self-harm. Find out if your youngster has a suicidal plan, if you can. The more specific the plan the greater the suicidal risk. A gun in the household may make it easy for your troubled teen to commit suicide. Nearly 60 percent of all suicides are committed with a firearm.

Providing Help

Although you may feel powerless, there are a number of things you can do to help a teen that is going through a difficult time. If you are concerned about your teen's behavior:

- Make sure your child has someone he or she can confide in. If your teen feels you don't understand, suggest a more neutral person—a grandparent, a priest or rabbi, a coach, a school counselor, or your child's doctor.
- Don't attempt to minimize or discount what your child is going through. This will only reinforce his or her sense of hopelessness.

- Always express your love, concern, and support.
- Don't postpone seeing a doctor. Your child should be evaluated for depression so that treatment can begin immediately.
- Express to your child that with help he or she will begin to feel better and his or her problems can be overcome.

Where to Find Help

If you think your child is suicidal, get help immediately. Your child's doctor can refer you to a psychologist or psychiatrist. Call your local hospital's department of psychiatry and ask for a list of doctors in your area. Your local mental health association or county medical society can also provide references. The warning signs for teen suicide are:

- A suicide threat or statement indicating a desire to die.
- A previous suicide attempt.
- Severe, prolonged depression.
- Marked changes in personality behavior, as in a sudden change from extremely depressed to extremely happy; a sudden change in friends; extreme changes in eating and sleeping habits; decreased academic performance; becoming very agitated; running away from home; or suddenly becoming irresponsible about such things as staying out late without telling parents.
- Making a will, giving away prized possessions, making final arrangements.

While these signs may seem obvious, they can be missed, misinterpreted, or not taken seriously. Teens will sometimes give warnings of an impending attempt by writing poetry or essays about suicide or about their death, and teachers are wise to alert the principal if they see this kind of writing. Suicidal teens are also likely to talk to a friend before they make an attempt, so it's important for your child to know what to do if a friend confides they are thinking about suicide. The rule of thumb any time you or your child hear talk of suicide from anyone is: No one should keep a secret about suicidal behavior.

> The rule of thumb any time you or your child hear talk of suicide from anyone is: No one should keep a secret about suicidal behavior.

If you believe your child is suicidal, you need to get professional help from a psychiatrist, psychologist, or counselor immediately. If the school is closed when you realize you need help, take your child to a hospital emergency room. The threat of suicide is too much for a parent to be dealing with on his or her own.

Vague references to suicide are sometimes made by teens. It is okay to follow up by asking directly about suicidal thoughts. Discussing suicide does not put thoughts of suicide in a person's head. On the contrary, it causes a realization that you are aware of the other person's feelings and thoughts. It can open the door to helping your adolescent know that he or she can be helped and is not alone.

After Suicide

Sometimes when a friend or classmate of your teen attempts or commits suicide, your adolescent may have many different emotions. Some teenagers say they feel guilty—especially the ones who feel they could have interpreted their friend's actions and words better. Others say they feel angry with the person who committed or attempted suicide for doing something so selfish. Still others say they feel nothing at all—they are too filled with grief. When someone attempts suicide, the people around him or her may feel afraid or uncomfortable about talking with him or her about it. If possible, your teen should try again to help; this is a time when a person absolutely needs to feel connected to others.

When someone commits suicide, the people around him or her may become very depressed and even think about suicide themselves. It's important for your adolescent to know that he or she should never blame themselves for someone's death. It's also good to know that any emotion your teen feels is appropriate; there is no right or wrong way to feel. Many schools will address the problem of a student's suicide head-on and call in special counselors to talk with students and help them deal with their feelings. If your adolescent is having difficulty dealing with a friend's or classmate's suicide, it's best to make use of these resources or talk to a trusted adult. Feeling grief after a friend commits suicide is normal. When it begins to interfere with everyday life, be sure your son or daughter is receiving counseling. Your school is the place to start for a referral.

EATING DISORDERS

The "ideal" body for women—the body seen on television, in advertisements and fashion magazines, in athletics, and in movies—can only be achieved by one percent of the population. This manufactured myth of the "perfect" body is often underweight and, in many cases, achieved through plastic surgery. Recent studies show that anywhere from four to 22 percent of college-age women report engaging in anorexic or bulimic behavior. In some cases, the disorder had gone undetected since high school or even middle school.

It is impossible to place all the blame for eating disorders on the media or society at large. One study did show that young women were strongly influenced by reading magazines depicting thin models and promoting thinness through dieting. Personality traits such as a need for control or a perfectionist attitude, wider concerns of family life or relationships outside the family, or even hereditary factors may also play a role in eating disorders.

Many of your daughters interpret the normal changes of puberty such as filling out of the thighs and breast development as getting fat. This may trigger dieting. The majority of teens who diet do not develop eating disorders. Additional factors such as sexual abuse, a death in the family, depression, and divorce can play a role in causing normal dieting to become a clinical eating disorder.

Types of Eating Disorders

Anorexia nervosa is a potentially life-threatening disorder in which a teen refuses to eat enough to maintain body weight that is normal for height. There is intense fear of gaining weight. Eventually menstruation—a young woman's period—stops. Teens with this disorder often strive for perfection and control over their lives by controlling their body weight. Typically, these teens see themselves as fat, even when most others see them as thin to the point of being ill. Dangerous weight loss behaviors, continual dieting, and simply refusing to eat are the hallmarks of this disorder.

Bulimia is a binge and purge syndrome. Teens suffering from bulimia frequently eat very large amounts of food followed by getting rid of the food by excessive physical activity, vomiting, or using laxatives. For bulimics, food is a source of comfort and security, and a barrier against insecurity or depression.

Binge eating may well be the most common eating disorder. In this case, binges are not followed by purges, and the person typically becomes obese. Binge eaters may lose great amounts of weight by dieting, sometimes up to 100 pounds, but usually regain the weight quickly if there is no change in how they view themselves and how they eat.

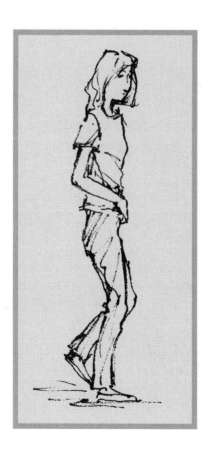

What Causes Eating Disorders?

Eating disorders are a serious signal that something is wrong. There is a whole set of underlying issues that must be identified and carefully considered. If left untreated, eating disorders can lead to obesity, skin irritations and deterioration, hair loss, and much worse, irreversible health damage such as stunted growth, thinning bones, damage to teeth and internal organs, and the inability to reproduce. Studies show that between 10 and 15 percent of young people with anorexia nervosa or bulimia die from complications of the disease.

Adults also need to know that teens with eating disorders are usually very secretive about their eating habits. Shame and guilt keep teens (and adults) from talking about an eating problem to the people they love the most. The most obvious signs of an eating disorder already well in progress are listed below.

- Eating in private, or having strange eating habits.
- Eating much less than usual and skipping meals.
- Loss of energy or serious fatigue.
- Light-headedness, dizziness, or fainting.
- Lack of physical growth.
- Loss of menstruation.
- Extreme weight loss or weight gain.
- Difficulty swallowing or keeping food down.
- Excessive tooth decay or loss of tooth enamel.
- Damage to the throat from repeatedly vomiting.

The following questions are designed to help you recognize an eating disorder before the disorder has advanced. If possible, discuss these questions with your teen. You may even wish to modify the questions to ask younger children, especially pre-teens just entering junior high or middle school. Yes answers to the questions below—whether based on your observations or told to you by your teen—indicate a possible eating disorder.

- Does your teen eat far less than usual or skip two or more meals a day?
- Does your teen want to eat alone or in private?
- Does your teen have new, seemingly strange eating habits?
- Does your teen eat a large amount of food within a two-hour period, often seeming out of control in eating?
- Does your teen eat large amounts of food when not hungry?
- Does your teen use laxatives, vomiting, excessive exercise, or other purging behavior to lose or control weight?
- Does your teen avoid social situations or stay at home to maintain an eating or exercise schedule?
- Does food seem to control your teen?
- Does your teen stay in the bathroom after meals taking a shower or with the water running? Are there signs of vomiting in the bathroom?
- Does your teen seem disgusted, depressed, or guilty after overeating?

Early Treatment Crucial

Given the seriousness of eating disorders and the secrecy that usually accompanies them, adults frequently need to be the first to seek help for their teen. The sooner an eating disorder is spotted and treatment is begun, the better the outlook. Experts recommend starting with the pediatrician or family physician. "It's important to do a physical exam to determine if the eating disorder has caused any physical harm and to rule out any other explanation for weight loss such as gastrointestinal or endocrine disorders," says Dr. Alexander R. Lucas, a child and adolescent psychiatrist at the Mayo Clinic. "Weight loss may also be due to depression in teens."

The next step is usually education about proper nutrition and psychotherapy while the adolescent remains at home. Counseling for the parents is also recommended. If the weight loss or binge eating and purging are out of control, hospitalization for more intensive treatment may be required. Please keep in mind that it is your teen daughter who must decide that she will handle her eating disorder and be well.

Real Hope: The Role of Sports, Exercise, and Activities

For some time now, our culture has promoted the idea that feminine beauty is associated with being lean, long-legged, and lithe. The pre-puberty body is looked

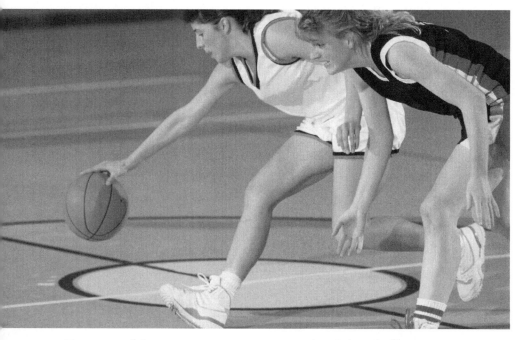

Team sports help young women to stay trim and to feel good about acquiring new skills and experiencing team camaraderie.

upon as ideal. Puberty with the redistribution of fat on your daughter's body makes this ideal figure impossible to attain for many girls.

There is hope for young women. That hope lies in their participation in athletics and in after-school activities. Athletics and exercise can benefit your daughter in many ways and should be strongly encouraged. First, team sports can keep weight off and contribute to a firmer, trimmer body. Second, with participation in sports, competence comes from mastering the skills and endurance needed. Young women feel good about themselves for their achievements, and so their mood is lifted. Developing team spirit and making friends helps, too. All the answers are not in yet about the positive effects of women and athletic involvement. Exactly how exercise affects mental health is not fully documented but enough data are available to be encouraging.

The same effect from participation in sports may well come from extra-curricular activities in school and in volunteering in the community. These activities increase a young woman's belief that she is worthwhile. She feels more positive about herself—for herself—not for her body shape.

However, a watchful eye is needed when young women become deeply involved in competitive sports. There is the potential for eating disorders to develop. In this situation, disorders are particularly difficult to deal with because body weight and composition may be factors in performance. Eating disorders can be life-threatening, and if they are added to the rigors of sports training without professional management, your son or your daughter can become at risk.

Learning Differences

What is ADHD?
Attention-Deficit Hyperactivity Disorder (ADHD) is a neuro-biological disorder marked by three distinct behaviors.

- INATTENTION—Not knowing what task to attend to or not being able to stay focused long enough to finish a task, and not being able to stay organized.
- IMPULSIVITY—Not being able to control urges to speak or act, and not thinking about the consequences.
- HYPERACTIVITY— Excess physical or mental restlessness, often without purpose or with a "driven" quality.

Dr. Russell Barkley, a leading authority who helps both professionals and families to understand ADHD, says that the three behaviors outlined above boil down to a problem with inhibition. That means if your adolescent has this disorder he or she may have trouble getting rid of the urge to do something else rather than the task at hand. There appears to be a delay in the development of the mental ability to wait in ADHD children and adolescents.

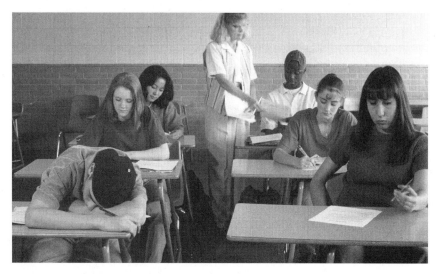

Adolescents with learning disabilities can feel very discouraged.
This chapter offers ideas to help these teens.

As humans, we learn to wait; this takes effort. In waiting, we separate our emotion from the information we have about a situation. We think about what happened in the past. We muse about what could happen in the future. We think about what would occur if we act in a certain way, or say certain words. We talk to ourselves and use that talk to control what we say and do. We may obtain new information and put it together with what we already know. We use this information to decide what to do. As Barkley says, if ADHD is a problem with a person's ability to inhibit response, we can't expect the person to work well in situations requiring being cool, calm, unemotional, or objective. Our society values these abilities with status, prestige, and even income.

> Barkley says, if ADHD is a problem with a person's ability to inhibit response, we can't expect the person to work well in situations requiring being cool, calm, unemotional, or objective.

On the other hand, those with ADHD may be very passionate and emotional in their responses. Barkley says that these children and adolescents may well match or surpass others in areas where using emotion is an advantage. Think about great musicians, poets, writers, and sales personnel, and how their passion serves them. Realize that those with ADHD respond very quickly—they don't leave time for using facts to guide their feelings.

Fortunately, says Barkley, medicine can produce the ability to inhibit and wait before responding. This helps those diagnosed with ADHD to behave and think much like others while they are taking medication. The individual has a chance to show self-control and free himself or herself from being controlled by the events of the moment.

While some 2 million school-age children have ADHD, this disorder frequently persists into adolescence and adulthood. Treatment for ADHD is based on individual needs, and may include special schooling, individual and/or family counseling, and medication. Support groups are also available. A professional skilled in working with the disorder should evaluate persons who exhibit the behavior patterns of ADHD. ADHD medications should be managed by physicians—typically psychiatrists, neurologists, and pediatricians specializing in development and behavior. Treatment for ADHD rarely includes medication alone.

How ADHD Affects the Community

Simply put, adolescents with ADHD don't do the things they mean to do—or say they will do—and they do things or say things that they don't mean to. Such a simple description may seem unfair to teens and adults already faced with the disorder, or may seem so general as to fit almost every adolescent. For some families, this simple description is a beginning toward looking at difficulties that may have been affecting a child and the whole family since the child was as young as three or four.

For adolescents with ADHD—diagnosed or undiagnosed—the disorder can spiral intro chronic behavior problems at school and at home, and lead to almost daily troubles with peers and authority figures. Adults often blame themselves for the disorder or think of their child as simply "bad." Besides the impact on families,

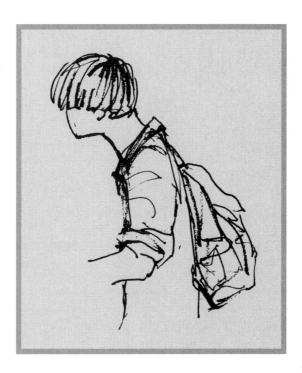

the social cost ripples outward into society in the form of lost productivity, under-employment, re-education costs, drug and alcohol abuse, and even crime.

What Parents Can Do

A summary of work from two important scholars in the area of ADHD indicates the importance of providing information to the parents and caregivers of ADHD adolescents.

In his encouraging book, *Taking Charge of ADHD*, Barkley urges parents to share his latest theory on ADHD—that the frontal part of the brain is where the mental process is located to stop or slow down behavior. He says the front part of the brain provides the power of self-control and the capacity to direct behavior toward the future. In other words, to think "what could happen if. ..."

Building on this theory, Barkley believes parents can accept their adolescent's disability and go about the business of helping to develop their self-control and advocate for the rights and services youngsters need.

This book has already presented a vivid word picture of the physical, emotional, and intellectual changes that occur during adolescence. These are normal changes that occur in the lives of adolescents. Adults are usually somewhat aware of the normal challenges of raising an adolescent. They certainly are after raising several adolescents.

In a family raising an ADHD adolescent, there is increased potential for academic failure, depression, loss of friends, poor self-esteem, addictive behaviors, and conflict at home. As Arthur Robin at Children's Hospital in Michigan says: "As long as an ADHD teen remains in your care, he or she is likely to require greater assistance from you than a non-ADHD teen does. While growing emotional maturity helps, the ADHD adolescent will lag behind other teens in developing self-control and organization."

> As Arthur Robin at Children's Hospital in Michigan says: "As long as an ADHD teen remains in your care, he or she is likely to require greater assistance from you than a non-ADHD teen."

Discussed below, very briefly, are Arthur Robin's suggestions for working with your ADHD adolescent. Refer to his chapter on adolescents in *Taking Charge of ADHD* for more information.

REASONABLE EXPECTATIONS. Expect your ADHD teen to:

- Achieve satisfactory grades.
- Follow basic family rules.
- Communicate without violence or temper outbursts.

These are expectations not demands, according to Robin. He says that you may interpret your adolescent's actions as a way to upset you—but ponder where that thinking gets you. Consider changing your thinking. What is worse, he proposes, losing face over a small issue or losing your relationship with your teen? Try hard to develop reasonable expectations and accurately look at your teen's actions.

Establishing, monitoring, and enforcing rules. Each family has bottom-line rules for living together and in the community. Some rules can be negotiated and some cannot. You will probably find that discussing the rules and making some compromises works better than simply setting up rules and expecting strict obedience.

Make a list of rules. Keep it short, and divide it into house and street rules, or however you think is easiest. Put the list in a prominent place and go over it frequently. Don't forget to discuss how all of us live by rules—this discussion makes rules for youngsters easier to follow.

As in any teen's home, your ADHD teen learns how to divide and conquer their parents. It is absolutely necessary to hold together as parents. An ADHD teen may need closer monitoring than other teens. Always know where your teen is. Be sure your adolescent lets you know his or her destination and any changes. Be up at curfew time. Monitor your ADHD teen's homework.

Systems of negative and positive consequences are used in the homes of many teens. Especially for the ADHD teen, the system needs to be backed up by a good deal of parental fortitude and no-nonsense attitude. You may have a very angry teen on your hands. Sometimes you may need the assistance of a therapist or even juvenile authorities.

Communication. Throughout this book there is an emphasis on positive communication. The same rules apply when you are conversing with your ADHD youngster. Raising that teen is sometimes so stressful that families resort to sarcasm, put downs, and accusations. Endless lectures end up with no behavioral change, and soon there is no conversation at all. Try to think through ways to improve the situation. For example, instead of tantrums (on either side) there can be counting to 10, taking a walk together, leaving the situation to cool down. Instead of commands there can be polite requests. Small mistakes can be overlooked. Practice and role-playing may seem downright silly, but it works. It is a lot better to try, than to endure a sullen teen who may be trying a good deal harder than you realize.

Problem-solving. Problem-solving models have long been taught in health education classes starting in elementary grades. If your ADHD teen has been taught this skill you can build on that experience. Teachers, social workers, and psychologists at your school can provide you an outline of how to proceed. Here is a school-based problem-solving outline:

1. Define the problem.
2. Discuss several solutions.
3. Evaluate the ideas and choose the best one.
4. Carry out the selected solution.
5. If the problem is not solved, go back to step 1.

Family problem-solving is not always easy. However, it is worth the effort. The exercise demands working together, avoiding getting mad or off the track, and restating the issues until everybody agrees. Sometimes a compromise must be reached. Look closely at what is blocking resolution toward agreement for your

ADHD teen—and for you. You can always get back to the problem the next week and try another solution.

You need to use a worksheet that follows a problem-solving outline. Remember to decide who will do what, when, where, and with what supervision. Clear cut consequences are very important for your teen to learn how to do, or how not to do, what is agreed upon.

Consequences should be written at the bottom of the problem-solving worksheet. Give your teen reminders during the week. Have everyone who is involved sign the bottom of the worksheet.

You can try this method over a period of time. Some families schedule regular family meetings. Along with planning for family vacations, visits to relatives, and assigning chores, a problem-solving worksheet can be used in these meetings. The chair person and secretary role can be alternated among family members. Good luck!

USE PROFESSIONAL HELP. ADHD expert Arthur Robin proposes establishing a relationship with a social worker, physician, or psychologist so that you can meet periodically to discuss progress for your ADHD young person. This preventive help can give you assistance before the going gets mired in conflict.

TAKE A VACATION. Maintain your sense of humor, says Dr. Robin. This too will pass, parents and caregivers learn. If you possibly can, be sure to plan a vacation from your ADHD adolescent several times a year. You'll recharge your batteries and come back fit to work with challenging parenting tasks.

WHAT IS DYSLEXIA?

According to the U.S. Department of Health and Human Services, it is estimated that as many as 15 percent of American students have dyslexia.

Research experts believe dyslexia is a change in the brain structure that causes individuals to have difficulty with the acquisition of language. As used here, dyslexia refers to a condition that causes individuals who exhibit average or above-average intelligence to have difficulty learning to read, write, spell, and process language.

People with dyslexia learn best when information is structured in a sequential fashion that moves from the simple to the complex.

The disorder is an impairment of the brain's ability to translate images received from the eyes into meaningful language. Although the basis of reading disability is unknown, there is evidence that it is caused by a malfunction of certain areas of the brain concerned with language.

Reading achievement significantly below that expected for age, is the key symptom of dyslexia. Dyslexia is not a disease. Nor is there a vaccination that will prevent it. Its causes are unclear. But dyslexia is not specific to age, gender, race, or ethnic background. The bad news is there is no cure for dyslexia. The good news is that dyslexia is a physiological or physical problem with an educational solution.

To most people, dyslexia simply means reading or writing backwards. However, people with dyslexia display a wide range of symptoms. Some adolescents with dyslexia remain poor spellers, for example, transposing letters within words, and adding letters, possibly because of poor auditory, visual, or phonic skills. Your adolescent may have an unusually short attention span, and have difficulty focusing on a task. Poor spatial skills and not being able to arrange material correctly may be a symptom.

It is hard to believe that in this day of instant communication, little information on dyslexia has reached the average parent, teacher, physician, psychologist, or others in positions to help. Yet successful teaching strategies have been in use for 60 years. Parents and caregivers need to become advocates in sharing with professionals. According to the National Institute for Health, only 10 percent of the teachers in our country are trained to teach students with dyslexia.

Dyslexia and school

Many teens with mild dyslexia are never identified, and therefore struggle through school. They may be described as "lazy," "not too bright," or "slow." The more severely affected students will be part of the bottom reading group and are often formally labeled "learning disabled." They frequently have feelings of being stupid or even retarded. Teachers sometimes tell them that if they would only try harder, listen better, and stay focused, they could succeed in their schoolwork. Dyslexia may be a condition that was overlooked in your teen's earlier school years. The following list of symptoms may help you determine if your son or daughter is dyslexic.

- Average to above average intelligence.
- Difficulty in sounding out unfamiliar words.
- Difficulty with memory and recall of words in written and oral expression.
- Comparatively high frequency of reading, writing, and spelling errors such as omissions, additions, substitutions, or reversals.
- Problems organizing, sequencing, and/or retrieving information.
- Difficulty following or remembering oral instructions.
- Reading, spelling and/or comprehension skills which fall below expectation.
- Excelling in art, music, drama, mechanics, problem-solving, or hands-on activities.

Related characteristics may include the following:

- Delayed speech development or speech problems.
- Left-handedness or ability to use both hands (ambidexterity).
- Family history of language learning problems.
- Difficulty in math.

- Allergies.
- Attention Deficit Disorder with or without hyperactivity.
- Difficulty with abstract concepts of time and direction (left-right confusion).

People with dyslexia learn best when information is structured in a sequential fashion that moves from the simple to the complex. Knowledge about language and its rules needs to be taught directly. For some, one-on-one instruction is essential. Seeing, saying, and doing (multi-sensory learning) is crucial. The first step in an instructional program is an approach called "synthetic phonics." The Orton-Gillingham teaching approach has been successful for thousands of people with dyslexia around the world.

Beyond Dyslexia

If a person with dyslexia fails often enough and is misunderstood, secondary emotional problems can arise which can further contribute to their difficulties. Many grow up with self-doubts about their intelligence and ability. Frustration and disappointment in their educational, occupational, and personal achievements are common.

If your dyslexic child's behavior has been carefully structured, he or she may not suffer any more than the normal stresses and strains common to all adolescents. For many dyslexic teens, however, adolescence is a difficult time. Often an adolescent will react in one of two ways. Some become hyperactive (because of an environmental overload of sights, sounds, and actions), and cannot focus on tasks. Others withdraw into themselves, spending most of their time daydreaming, at home and in school.

Parents and teachers must be alert and attempt to identify these individuals. Both types of dyslexic adolescents, the hyperactive and the withdrawn, can be helped. Everyone needs to feel good about himself or herself. One of the biggest problems for the dyslexic adolescent is that mistakes take away the opportunity to discover strengths.

Both parents and teachers must give dyslexic adolescents a sense that they are important, by affirming a positive perception of who they are and how they can make their lives happier. By working together, the family and the school can help a dyslexic adolescent change poor self-perception from "I can't succeed," to "I can make it," "I will try," and "I can succeed."

Organizational skills

The day-to-day strain of the numerous tasks requiring attention, organization, planning, and remembering makes your adolescent with dyslexia resist the reward of independence and self-sufficiency. You or your teen's teachers need to introduce strategies for helping to cope with those tasks that demand organization and social interaction.

One of the best strategies is to encourage the dyslexic adolescent to make up checklists outlining each step of a particular task.

Below are some additional strategies for daily survival that help your adolescent with dyslexia learn organizational skills. Teach your dyslexic adolescent to:

- Read and follow a recipe.
- Set the table correctly.
- Make a shopping list, estimate the amount of money needed, and make choices.
- Read a menu, understand the check, estimate the tip, and pay the bill.
- Count, make change, keep an account, and use a budget.
- Make a schedule for activities, dates, appointments, household chores, shopping, and school.
- Remember the home telephone number and emergency numbers, plus how to dial numbers, answer the telephone politely, and ask pertinent questions.

Remember your dyslexic adolescent often needs much more time to complete tasks and also requires additional time between difficult tasks. A dyslexic teen may suffer greatly from fatigue because he or she must concentrate fiercely in order to think in an organized way.

You need a great deal of patience to treat the adolescent dyslexic with understanding and love. Both you and your teen's teachers should not set unrealistic goals. Treating a dyslexic teen like a child just won't work. The adolescent dyslexic needs to be supported every step of the way and yet still be encouraged to be as independent as possible.

With family support and proper teaching, students with dyslexia can succeed in all walks of life. Many dyslexics excel in architecture, music, interior decorating,

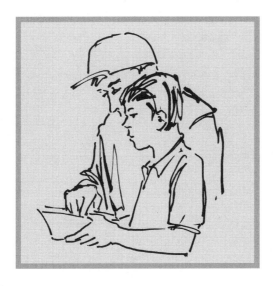

engineering, the arts, business, politics, painting, poetry, and prose. They often like and are good at hands-on activities.

If your teenager has many characteristics from the checklists, you may want to look into testing for dyslexia by a trained specialist in that field. It could be a psychologist, a physician, or a language evaluator for dyslexia. If your school has no specially trained teachers available, look for outside help. There are organizations that can put you in touch with help in your area (see the resource list at the end of this chapter). Communicate the results of the testing to your teen's teachers to make them aware of your teen's strengths and weaknesses. By law, if a person is diagnosed with dyslexia, they have the right to certain accommodations and instruction. Inquire about untimed tests, oral examinations, and even bringing a tape recorder into the classroom. Keep in mind that the need for untimed tests must be documented prior to taking these tests. Teens with dyslexia can also take the ACT and SAT tests orally. You can help by giving practice tests so your son or daughter can develop test-taking abilities.

The dyslexic adolescent may have difficulty establishing relationships because of distorted interpretations of the feelings of others. He or she may also have trouble reading facial expressions and communicating appropriately. Dyslexic adolescents who grow up feeling unworthy, stupid, or lonely, have warped perceptions of themselves. Developing relationships is the adolescent's most important task. You, as the parent or caregiver need to put more energy into helping a dyslexic son or daughter become a successful and contributing adult.

Central Auditory Processing Disorder

Another consideration for school inefficiency is a Central Auditory Processing Disorder (CAPD), which results in behaviors similar to Attention Deficit Disorder. The student with CAPD has normal peripheral hearing sensitivity, however, he or she has a reduced ability to discriminate, recognize, or comprehend auditory information. When the acoustic environment is less than ideal, the student may not hear bits and pieces of lectures, discussions, and essential facts.

Some associated behaviors include:

- Frequent misunderstanding of oral instructions.
- Delay in responding to questions.
- Need for directions to be repeated.
- Frequent response of "What?" or "Huh?"
- Difficulty in understanding when there is background noise.
- Possible academic problems involving spelling or reading.
- An overall appearance of looking disinterested, unfocused, not paying attention.

If you think that these behaviors fit your teen, an audiologist with the correct equipment can diagnose this problem. It is important to sort out what the problem is and what it is not, since CAPD can cause significant problems in a teen's academic life.

REFERENCES AND RESOURCES

Please refer to the references and resources section of Chapter One for many books related to developing a mentally healthy adolescent.

Stress

Coping with Stress, Gwen Packard (Hazelden/Rosen, 1997, $6.95). Advice for teens on de-stressing.

Fighting Invisible Tigers: A Stress Management Guide for Teens, Earl Hipp (Free Spirit Publishing, 1995, $10.95). Proven, practical advice for teens on coping with stress, being assertive, taking risks, making decisions, staying healthy, dealing with fears, building relationships, and more.

Mind Over Mood: Change How You Feel by Changing the Way You Think, Dennis Greenburger and Christine A. Padesky (The Guilford Press, 1995, $21.00). A hands-on workbook for people suffering from depression, panic attacks, anxiety, eating disorders, substance abuse, and relationship problems. Includes case examples, written exercises, and clear step-by-step instructions.

Taking Charge of My Mind & Body: A Girls' Guide to Outsmarting Alcohol, Drugs, Smoking, and Eating Problems, G. Folkers and J. Engelmann (FreeSpirit Publishing, 1998, $13.95). A friendly book about making healthy choices.

Teenage Stress, Daniel Cohen and Susan Cohen (M. Evans and Co, 1984, $19.50). Written at a young adult reading level, this book discusses stress and its causes, what it does to and for one, and how to keep life stress at a tolerable level.

Depression

American Academy of Child and Adolescent Psychiatry, 202-966-7300. Web site: www.aacap.org.

Conversations at The Carter Center: Coping with the Stigma of Mental Illness (video), hosted by Rosalynn Carter; narrated by Joanne Woodward (27 minutes, The Carter Center Mental Health Program, One Copenhill, Atlanta, GA 30307, 404-420-5165, $12.00, requests for free copies considered). Author Kathy Cronkite and actor Rod Steiger discuss their personal experiences coping with mental illness and then answer questions from a live audience. Treatments are discussed.

Darkness Visible: A Memoir of Madness, by William Styron (Vintage Books, 1992, $10.00). Styron writes about his experience with depression as only a master of words can—he allows us to enter his mind with compelling honesty. Careful reading of this short volume will not only advance your empathy for those who are mentally ill, but will help you to understand how devastating that unseen illness can be.

Depression and Related Affective Disorders Association (DRADA), (410-955-4647. John Hopkins Hospital Meyer 3-181, 600 N. Wolfe, Baltimore MD 21287. Web site: www.med.jhu.edu/jhhpsychiatry/affective.htm).

A Family Guide to Systems of Care for Children with Mental Health Needs, (CMHS National Mental Health Services, Knowledge Exchange Network, 800-789-2647. Web site: www.mentalhealth.org/child.) Intended to assist parents and caregivers who are seeking help for children with mental health problems. Bilingual (Spanish and English) information guide includes what they need to know, ask, expect, and do to get the most out of care.

Helping Your Depressed Teenager: A Guide for Parents and Caregivers, Gerald D. Oter and Sarah S. Montgomery (John Wiley & Sons, 1994, $23.95). Covers teen development, understanding depression, and how to help your teen.

Helpline (suicide and depression): 800-852-3388

How to Cope with Depression—A Complete Guide for You and Your Family, J. Raymond DePaulo Jr., and Keith R. Ablow (Ballantine Books, 1996, $10.00). Two physicians present depression from four perspectives: Disease, personality, behavior, and life stories.

Life Happens: A Teenager's Guide to Friends, Failure, Sexuality, Love, Rejection, Addiction, Peer Pressure, Families, Loss, Depression, and Change, Charles Wibbelsman, M.D., and Kathy McCoy (Perigee, 1996, $11.00).

Lonely, Sad and Angry: A Parent's Guide to Depression in Children and Adolescents, Barbara D. Ingersoll and Sam Goldstein (Main Street Books, 1996, $12.95). The authors define depression in straightforward terms and explain how depression differs from the normal "ups and downs" of life. Explains how parents can recognize warning signs, and outlines the various medical, psychological, and environmental causes and treatments.

Lost and Found, (Film Ideas, 1996, $150.00, 22 minutes). This is a Children's Hospital of Michigan video featuring eight adolescents, ages 12-20, who have been depressed. Outstanding consultation on this video from Dr. J.P. Leleszi, Director of Consultation and Pediatric Hospice at Wayne State University.

National Alliance for the Mentally Ill, (703-524-7600, 800-950-6264 helpline) 200 N. Glebe Rd. Suite 1015, Arlington VA 22203-3754. Web site: www.nami.org.

National Depressive and Manic-Depressive Association, (800-826-3632, 312-642-0049. 730 N. Franklin, Suite 501, Chicago, IL 60610. Web site: www.ndmda.org). Offers mail-order bookstore on depression. Write for a free catalog.

National Foundation for Depressive Illness, Inc., (800-245-4305, 212-268-4260, PO Box 2257, NY, NY 10116). Information and a list of physicians who specialize in affective disorders.

National Institute of Mental Health, (800-421-4211, 5600 Fishers Lane Rm. 10-85, Parklawn Bldg., Rockville MD 20857, Web site: www.nimh.nih.gov). Offers free brochures on depression.

National Mental Health Association, (800-969-6642, 1021 Prince Street Alexandria VA 22314-2971. Web site: www.nmha.org).

National Youth Crisis Hotline: 800-448-4663, 800-448-1833 TDD. A 24-hour crisis line for any crisis.

Now We Can Successfully Treat the Illness Called Depression, National Foundation for Depressive Illness, Inc. (P.O. Box 2257 New York, NY 10116, free). Defines depressive illnesses and describes treatment options. Other booklets available.

Recovery Inc., (312-337-5661, 802 N. Dearborn St., Chicago, IL 60610). Self-help group to identify self-defeating and illness promoting thoughts and impulses and replace them with self-endorsing thoughts and actions. Write for a group near you.

The Romance of Risk: Why Teenagers Do the Things They Do, Lynn E. Poynton (Basic Books, 1998, $14.00). A leading figure in adolescent psychiatry presents the direct stories of 15 troubled adolescents, to explain the natural tendency of teenagers toward risk-taking. Suggests ways that parents can redirect this natural impulse into healthy and safe channels.

Teenline. 800 639-6095.

Understanding Depression: A Complete Guide to Its Diagnosis & Treatment, Donald F. Klein and Paul H. Wender (Oxford University Press, 1994, $9.95). A definitive guide to depressive illness—its causes, course, and symptoms.

Suicide

American Association of Suicidology, Web site: www.suicidology.org.

American Foundation for Suicide Prevention, 888-333-AFSP, Web site: www.afsp.org.

American Suicide Foundation, 212 363-3500, 120 Wall St. NY NY 10005.

Infoline for Suicide Help, 800-203-1234, Web site: www.infoline.org.

National Suicide Referral, 202 237-2280.

No One Saw My Pain: Why Teens Kill Themselves, Andrew Slaby and Lili Frank Garfinkel (W.W. Norton & Company, 1994, $12.00). Slaby, a psychiatrist specializing in depression and crisis intervention, found that the severity of distress in teens was missed because people didn't know what to look for.

The Power to Prevent Suicide: A Guide for Teens Helping Teens, Richard E. Nelson and Judith C. Galas (Free Spirit Publishing, 1994, $11.95). How to recognize the warning signs, reach out to friends at risk, and get help.

SA/VE, Suicide Awareness/Voices Education, 612-946-7998, Web site: www.save.org.

Suicide Prevention Hotline, 800-827-7571.

Suicide Prevention Resources, 212-459-2611.

Suicide: Why? Adina Wrobleski (Afterwords, 1995, $12.95). Addresses 85 questions about suicide.

When A Friend Dies: A Book for Teens About Grieving and Healing, Marilyn E. Gootman, (Free Spirit, 1994, $7.95).

Gentle advice for any teen who is grieving the death of a friend.

When Nothing Matters Any More: A Survival Guide for Depressed Teens, by Bev Cobain (Free Spirit, 1998, $13.95). Bev Cobain knows about feeling "beyond blue" from personal experience—she has survived the suicides of three members of their family, including Kurt, her superstar cousin. This book gives teens the information and encouragement they need to recognize depression, realize they don't need to live in pain, and most importantly, tells them how to get help.

Eating Disorders

Academy for Eating Disorders. (703-556-9222, 703-556-8729-fax. 6728 Old McLean Village Drive, McLean, VA 22101-3906. E-mail address: aed@degnon.org. Web site: www.acadeatdis.org).

Afraid to Eat: Children and Teens in Weight Crisis, Frances M. Berg (Healthy Weight Press, $17.95, www.healthyweightnetwork.com). Documents the profound mental and physical damage to children and teens caused by America's obsession with weight and being thin. Gives caring adults clear guidelines on how to make needed changes—at home, in school, and even in the wider culture. Preview and order online.

American Anorexia/Bulimia Association, Inc. (AABA), (212-575-6200, E-mail address: AmAnBu@aol.com, Web site: members.aol.com/AmAnBu). Information on eating disorders, referrals to clinics, hospital programs and support groups.

Anorexia Nervosa and Related Eating Disorders, Inc. (ANRED), (541-344-1144, P.O. Box 5102, Eugene, Oregon 97405, E-mail address: jarinor@rio.com, Web site: www.anred.com).

Eating Disorders (free); *Eating for Life* ($1.00); *Food Allergies: Rare but Risky* (free); *Should You Go On a Diet?* (for teens—free). Write to R. Woods, Consumer Information Center - 6A-2, P.O. Box 100, Pueblo, Colorado 81002 for these publications and/or a complete catalog of available publications. Internet Web address: http://www.pueblo.gsa.gov.

Hunger Pains: The Modern Woman's Tragic Quest for Thinness, Mary Pipher (Ballantine Books, 1997, $10.00). From a leading author and therapist.

National Association of Anorexia Nervosa and Associated Disorders (ANAD), (847-831-3438, E-mail address: anad20@aol.com). Free information, telephone counseling and nationwide referrals to therapists, support groups, and physicians.

Real Gorgeous: The Truth About Body & Beauty, Kaz Kooke (W.W. Norton, 1996, $13.00). A good, hard look at how girls and women have been mislead to think they should look like a model. Kaz Kooke uses her great sense of humor, funny chapter titles, and illustrations to make her point: each of us is special in her own way. Good reading for boys and men, as well.

Straight Talk About Eating Disorders, Michael Maloney and Rachel Kranz (Facts on File, 1991, $19.95). Offers clear information on different types of eating disorders, including bulimia and anorexia, examines the contradictory messages that teens receive about diet and appearance, and explains how to get help and support.

Women's Sports Foundation, (800-227-3988, Eisenhower Park, East Meadow, NY 11554). Provides information on eating disorders, physical fitness, the female athlete, exercise, and drugs.

Learning Differences

1100 Words You Need to Know, Murray Bromberg and Melvin Gordon (Barron's Educational Series, 1993, $10.95). A 46-week program to increase critical, commonly used vocabulary. Good for those with dyslexia. Excellent preparation for ACT and SAT tests and college-level reading.

1997-1998 Directory of Facilities and Services for the Learning Disabled, (17th edition: Academic Therapy Publications, 20 Commercial Blvd, Novato, CA 94949-6191). Copies available at no charge; requests should include a $5.00 postage/handling fee for each copy.

About Dyslexia: Unraveling The Myth, Priscilla Vail (Modern Learning Press, 1990, $6.95). A book of insight into the strengths and weaknesses of people with dyslexia.

ADHD and Teens: A Parent's Guide to Making It Through the Tough Years, Colleen Alexander-Roberts (Taylor Publishing, 1995, $12.95). Teens with ADHD have an extremely high risk of school and social problems which can lead to academic failure and disruptive family relationships. Practical advice.

ADHD In Adolescence: Diagnosis, Arthur Robin (Gillford Press, 1998, $48.95). Book for physicians, psychologists, educators, knowledgeable parents, for diagnosing and treating ADHD in the second decade of life.

ADHD Lifespan Center, (Wayne State University, Detroit Medical Center, Children's Hospital, 313-745-4882). For all ages. Diagnosis, psychological testing and therapy, education, medication, and school advocacy.

All About Attention Deficit Disorder: Symptoms, Diagnosis and Treatment: Children and Adults, Thomas W. Phelan (Child Management, 1996, $12.95, audio cassette for $24.95). Presented with warmth and intelligence, this comprehensive guide gives parents, teachers, pediatricians, and mental health professionals the facts and resources they need to effectively deal with ADD.

Attention Deficit Disorder: A Different Perception, Thom Hartmann (Underwood Books, 1997, $12.00). Provides an inside view of how people with ADD think and function in society.

Attention Deficit Disorder Association, (8091 South Ireland Way, Aurora, CO 80016, 303-690-7548).

Attention Deficit Disorder Warehouse, (800-233-9273, E-mail address: sales@warehouse.com, Web site: www.addwarehouse.com). Many of the listed books are available.

Beaumont Center for Human Development (Royal Oak, MI, 248-691-4744). Evaluation services, tutoring, and counseling.

Children and Adults with Attention Deficit Disorders (CHADD), (800-233-4050, Web site: www.chadd.org). Parents/professionals: How to organize support groups, information on conferences and chapters.

Council for Exceptional Children: Eric Clearinghouse on Disabilities and Gifted Children, (800-328-0272. Web Site: http://ericec.org).

Driven to Distraction: Recognizing and Coping with Attention Deficit Disorder from Childhood through Adulthood, Edward M. Hallowell and John J. Ratey (Simon & Schuster, 1995, $13.00). Two doctors offer a readable, useful book on ADHD. Stories from child and adult sufferers.

Dyslexia: Background for an Action Agenda for Teacher Training, John C. Howell (available at the Dyslexia Store, see listing below, $5.00). A must read for teachers, school administrators, and parents. Clear, concise, and compelling, Dr. Howell answers your questions regarding dyslexia.

Dyslexia Store, Michigan Dyslexia Institute/Dyslexia Association of America, (532 E. Shiawassee Street, Lansing, MI 48912-1214, 800-495-6758, 517-485-4076 fax, Web site: www.dyslexia.net). Carries extensive line of books on dyslexia and learning disabilities. Free catalog.

Eton Transition Center, (Birmingham, Michigan, 248-642-1150, E-mail address: etonac.aol.com). Individualized curriculum for learning disabled students. Recognized as a school of excellence by the U.S. Department of Education in 1999.

Help for the Learning Disabled Child: Symptoms and Solutions, Lou Stewart (Slosson Educational Publications, 800-828-4800, 1990, $29.95). Aid to parents and professionals. Confirms learning disabled and ADHD symptoms and provides methods to use.

Helping Your Dyslexic Child, by Ellen Cronin (Prima Publishing, 1994, $13.00). The author of this book has studied dyslexia for many years and has developed a working program that parents can use to help dyslexic children significantly improve their reading, writing, and spelling. Beginning with a simple test that you can conduct at home, Cronin presents a comprehensive and holistic program that any parent or teacher can easily use.

Keeping A Head in School: A Student's Book About Learning Disabilities and Learning Disorders, Mel Levine (Educators Publishing Services and ADD Warehourse, 1991, $22.00). The book helps youngsters age 9-15 who have learning problems better understand their personal strengths and weaknesses. Dr. Mel Levine is a pediatrician and well-known authority on learning problems.

A Layman's Look at Dyslexia, Ronald E. Weger (available at the Dyslexia Store, see listing above, 1989, $10.00). Covers dyslexia from statistics to individual triumphs. Easy reading.

Living with a Learning Disability, Barbara Cordoni (Southern Illinois University Press, 1991, $17.95). Social barriers can cause more of a loss of self-esteem and personal pain than academic proficiency.

Making the Grade: An Adolescent's Struggle with ADD with Commonly Asked Questions & Answers About ADD, Roberta N. Parker and Harvey C. Parker (Specialty Press, Inc., 1992, $11.00). This is a heart-warming story of seventh grader Jim Jerome's struggle to succeed in school. In Commonly Asked Questions, symptoms, causes, treatments, and outcomes of ADD are discussed frankly and positively.

National Center for Learning Disabilities, (381 Park Avenue South, Suite 1420, New York, NY 10016, 212-545-7510. Web Site: www.ncld.org).

A National Directory of Four-Year Colleges, Two-Year Colleges, and Post-High School Training Programs for Young People with Learning Disabilities, P.M. Fielding (Partners in Publishing, 1993, $29.95).

Solve Your Child's School-Related Problems, Michael Martin and Cynthia Waltman-Greenwood (Harper Collins, 1995, $18.00). A guide for concerned parents provides insight into current development theories while offering solutions to more than 70 common problems that children face in school, including ADHD and drug abuse.

The Survival Guide for Teenagers with LD (Learning Differences), Rhoda Cummings and Gary Fisher (Free Spirit Publishing, 1996, $11.95, audio tape $19.95). Clear, comprehensive, and matter-of-fact, this guide helps teens with LD succeed in school and prepare for life as adults.

Surviving Public School: A Guide for Parents of Learning Disabled (Dyslexic) Kids, Thomas W. Conwell (available at the Dyslexia Store, see listing above, 1994, $10.00). A step-by-step plan for not only surviving public school, but winning the war for your child.

Taking Charge of ADHD, Russell A. Barkley (Guilford Press, New York, 1995, $17.95). Provides comprehensive, up-to-date information and expert advice on managing children and adolescents with ADHD. Dr. Barkley's ideas and theories are summarized in the text of *Healthy Teens* (with permission), as is the work of Dr. Arthur Robin related to teens.

Teenagers with ADD: A Parents' Guide, Chris A. Ziegler Dendy (Woodbine House, 1995, $18.95). Gives parents necessary tools to raise a healthy teen with positive attitudes.

What Every Teacher and Parent Should Know About Dyslexia, Dave Sargent and Laura Tirella (Ozark Publishing, 1996, $29.95). Questions and answers, suggestions for parents and modifications for teachers.

What You Need To Know about Ritalin, James Shaya, James Windell and Holley Gilbert (Bantam, 1999, $6.50). A definitive guide that parents, caregivers, and professionals need in understanding Ritalin. Thoughtful work by well-qualified authors with excellent credentials.

CHAPTER 4
TEEN SEXUALITY

This chapter presents an overview of issues parents and caregivers need to consider as they discuss sexuality with their teen. It includes explicit material about sexually transmitted diseases including the human immunodeficiency virus (HIV).

TEENS: HEARING FROM PARENTS

Teens want to hear more from their parents about sex, values, and relationships, according to James Jaccard, Ph.D., Distinguished Professor at the State University of New York in Albany, who has studied information from 20,000 students in grades 7 through 12.

Contrary to popular expectations, kids care about what adults think, even though parents and other adults often say they feel awkward discussing sex and relationships with teens, that they are not sure what to say, or that teens do not listen anyway.

"Don't nag or lecture," says Dr. Jaccard, a researcher with the National Longitudinal Study of Adolescent Health (Add Health Study). "Listen to what your adolescent has to say with an open mind. Express your feelings and expectations."

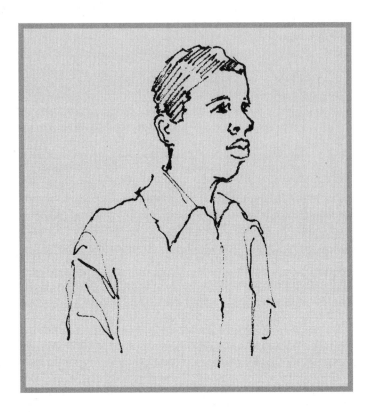

Dr. Jaccard outlines central facts in communicating with teens about sexual activity. These are:

- Parents and caregivers tend to underestimate the sexual activity of their children. They may talk to their children about sexual issues at around 12 years of age, but statistics show that a number of children are sexually active at this age. It is important to talk about sexuality before your child becomes sexually active.

- Most parents and caregivers dread the "big talk." They are glad when it is over and they are finished. As this book has consistently pointed out, an 11-year-old and a 16-year-old are very different young people. The kinds of issues parents need to be addressing are different as adolescents mature.

- Adults talking to their children about sexual activity will do so using their own value system. If parents and caregivers talk about a broad range of reasons for not engaging in sexual-risk behavior, they will be more successful than dwelling on just pregnancy or sexually transmitted diseases. This reasoning can include religious, moral, social, and emotional issues to motivate young people not to engage in risky sexual behavior. Adults can discuss how teen pregnancy can destroy life planning. They can carefully outline why their religion does not condone pre-marital sex. Frankness about the effort and expense of raising children can be pursued. Another consideration is to talk about what positive benefits your teen sees in engaging in risky behavior. If a boyfriend or girlfriend is pushing for sexual activity, what does this say about a relationship?

- Too often, adults turn discussions into one way lectures. This will not work with adolescents. Communication, in this area as in every other area with your adolescent, should be honest, open, and respectful. Each side needs to listen to the other.

- Parents and caregivers need to be sure that discussions about sexuality and sexual activity are held in a quiet place, free of interruption and stress. It is not a good idea to combine tasks with this kind of discussion.

- Adolescents who say they know all there is to know about sexual issues do not know any more than other teens. Statements such as "I know everything" should be disregarded; parents and caregivers must take responsibility for providing helpful information.

- For adults who know that their child is sexually active, who discover that their daughter is pregnant, that their unmarried son is a father, or that their teen has HIV, the issues are complex. Parents who experience having children who take risks that produce these consequences often blame themselves. They have a range of emotions including disappointment, anger, and sadness. This is normal. At such a time it is important to remain as cool as possible and to use these problem-solving strategies: define the problem; carefully discuss options; seek community resources; and evaluate your direction. It is a time to do away with ranting and anger, and to be supportive about a difficult life experience for a son or daughter. Practical suggestions include further serious discussions about the value of abstinence and family values. Providing contraceptive information, seeking medical services and treatment are important. Working together on problem-solving will be challenging. However, a child who runs away from home, who seeks solace in drugs or commits suicide, presents another set of problems, and deeper sorrow.

Dangers of Ignorance and Fear

There are numerous myths about sex, sexuality, and sexually transmitted diseases. Be sure to address each of these issues with your child. Ask your son or daughter to explain to you their views and beliefs about each of these areas, and encourage them to be specific and detailed. Create an environment in which they feel emotionally secure to share with you. There will be no effective communication with your preteen or teen unless you have their trust and respect. When listening, it is important that you do not appear to be judgmental or aghast at their responses. If

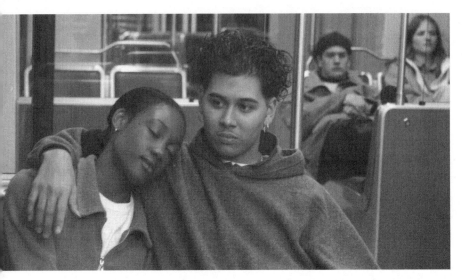

*Have adults prepared these young people how to be physically
and emotionally safe and responsible to one another?*

these topics of discussion are very difficult for you, then perhaps there is a friend
or family member whom you trust and who has a good rapport with your child.
Remember, each child eventually seeks answers to their own questions; it is best if
those answers come from you or a trusted relative or friend.

Adolescents often do not connect their actions with consequences. More
than 74 percent of today's teens engage in sexual activities before they graduate
from high school. Every year, 1.2 million adolescents become pregnant and 2.5
million acquire sexually transmitted diseases, despite the best efforts of parents,
teachers, and others in the community.

When young people look to television for answers and direction, they do
not find it in the four to six hours they watch on average each day. Over one-half
of all shows and two-thirds of prime time shows have sexual content. A sparse
nine percent include references to safer sex, contraception or abstinence, according
to a study conducted by the Kaiser Family Health Foundation. Of 88 scenes
involving sexual intercourse, none made reference to the risks—pregnancy, depression or disease.

When discussing abstinence and teenage parenthood, a budget exercise has
proven to be an extremely useful tool. Ask your teen to list and estimate the cost
of all the expenses of having a baby and raising a child. This forces the teen to actually visualize life as it could be, and reaffirms the difficulty with teenage parenting.

Sister Souljah, a rap singer and novelist, says the main thing that counts with
children and adolescents is their parent's consistent presence. "In America most
people spend the majority of time in pursuit of survival; kids are left to design their
lives for themselves, and most of them do that very chaotically."

All too often, peers and television become the source of reference. Parents and caregivers who make sex education an ongoing process—something normal to discuss—can save themselves and their teens from the awkward, one-time, big deal conversation about sex. They might even save their teen's life.

What to Tell Teens

The following guidelines come from the American Academy of Pediatrics regarding what to tell teens about sex. Well before they reach their early teens, both boys and girls should already know:

- The basics of sexual "plumbing," that is, the names and functions of male and female sex organs.
- The purpose and meaning of puberty (moving into young womanhood or young manhood).
- The function of the menstrual cycle (period).
- What sexual intercourse is and how women become pregnant.

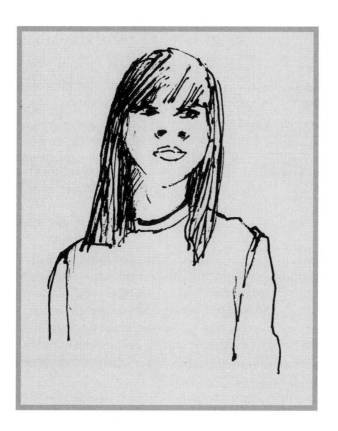

Once your child becomes a teenager, the focus of your talks about sex should shift. You should begin to talk to your teen about the social and emotional aspects of sex, and about your values. You will want to deal with issues that help your teenager answer questions like these:

- "When should I start dating?"
- "When is it okay to kiss a boy (or a girl)?"
- "How far is too far?"
- "How will I know when I'm ready to have sex?"
- "Won't having sex help me keep my boyfriend (or girlfriend)?"

Used with permission of the American Academy of Pediatrics, *"Talking to Your Young Teen About Sex and Sexuality: Guidelines for Parents,"* 1997.

Everywhere the researchers for the National Campaign to Prevent Teen Pregnancy went, the teens told them they want to hear more from their parents about sex, values, and relationships. Contrary to popular opinion, kids care about what adults think. Even though you might be uneasy about your conversation, you should not stop trying to communicate. You can always say, "I am uncomfortable with this discussion, but please know how important I believe it is." Be very clear about your values.

The more you listen to what your teen is saying, the greater chance of keeping lines of communication open. You can provide your teen with some of the materials recommended in our REFERENCES AND RESOURCES section at the end of this chapter.

Become aware of the world your teen lives in. Talk to a friend, buy some teen magazines, and visit your public library. Read as much as you can about teen sexuality and be prepared to be open and honest in your conversations. Go to school and read the health lessons offered to middle school and high school students. Follow up with your student's teacher if you have any questions about the lessons. Join with your school in seeing to it that positive, constructive, thorough, information is taught.

Make sure that your teen knows the facts about pregnancy and sexually transmitted diseases including HIV and AIDS.

Help your teen understand the internal and external pressures to express their sexuality and to make responsible decisions. In other words, your teen needs to know where you stand. You need to share your hopes for your teen's future as well as your concerns for the day-to-day issues your teen might be facing. Bear in mind that you do not own your child, nor control his or her thinking. You can influence your teen's decisions but cannot make decisions for him or her.

Make sure that your teen knows the facts about pregnancy and sexually transmitted diseases including HIV and AIDS. If you cannot provide information yourself, find someone who can, and ask him or her to talk with your teen. Check the REFERENCES AND RESOURCES section at the end of this chapter for information. Most importantly, find out when, how, and how much information about

HIV your student is learning at school. In many states, HIV education is mandated by law; the quantity and quality of the education varies.

Try to be available to your teen, no matter what. Teens tend to live for today. Discussions you and your teens have, and decisions you make together, will be tested by time and events in your teen's life. It is a good idea to be realistic about the fears and pressures your teens face on a daily basis. The environment today is faster-paced and perhaps more dangerous than when you were a teen. Sometimes teens are more capable intellectually than they are emotionally. Let them know you will always be there. Listen to them when they need help, without judging or criticizing them for getting stuck in their thinking. Your help in an emotional crisis could lead to lasting awareness.

Smart Parenting Works Wonders

What can parents do to prevent teens from experimenting with behavior that puts them at risk? Researchers Kim S. Miller Ph.D. and Daniel Whitaker Ph.D., from the Centers for Disease Control and Prevention's (CDC's) Division of HIV/AIDS Prevention, recently interviewed 907 adolescents and their mothers in the Bronx; San Juan, Puerto Rico; and Montgomery, Alabama, to find out how mother-child communications about sex relates to adolescents' sexual behavior. Here are some pointers from their discussion:

- Mothers who were skilled communicators about sex-related topics were more likely to discuss a broad range of issues with their adolescents and more likely to be heard by them. Teens appreciated mothers who had accurate information, who talked openly and freely rather than lecturing them, and who listened to the adolescents' own concerns and feelings about the topic.

- When mothers discussed a full range of sexual issues, adolescents engaged in less risky sexual behavior.

- Adolescents who talked with their mothers before their first sexual encounter were three times more likely to use a condom than were those who did not talk to their mothers. Adolescents who used condoms the first time they had intercourse were 20 times more likely to use condoms regularly in subsequent acts.

- Avoiding discussions about sex can lead adolescents to rely on their peers. This can be a problem if peers do not encourage responsible behavior such as abstinence or using a condom.

- The predictors of mothers and daughters talking included the mother having information and being comfortable about talking about condoms.

As researchers Miller and Whitaker say when discussing the role of families in *Adolescent HIV Risk Prevention: The Role of the Family*:

Many experts agree that it is the parents who are the most powerful socializing agents in the lives of young teens. Parents and other adults are in a unique and powerful position to shape young people's attitudes and behaviors, and to socialize them to become healthy adults. They do this in part by providing accurate information about risks, consequences, and responsibilities, and by imparting skills to make responsible decisions about health. However, the strength of their impact, relative to other information sources, may arise from their unique ability to engage their children in dialogues about development and decision making which are continuous (i.e., not one-time events), sequential (i.e., building one upon the next as the child's cognitive, emotional, physical, and social development and experiences change), and time-sensitive (i.e., information is immediately responsive to the child's questions and anticipated needs rather than programmed, such as in a school curriculum).

Reprinted with permission from Kim S. Miller, Ph.D., 1999.

Head Off Trouble

Sexual activity can result in pregnancy or sexually transmitted diseases. Some of the early indicators of trouble include:

> Helping your teen develop a strong sense of self, high self-esteem, and a compelling belief in respectable values and ethical behavior are the best things you can do to prevent irresponsible sexual behavior.

EARLY DATING: The likelihood of teen pregnancy and of sexually transmitted diseases is much greater for teens who start to date before the age of 14 or 15. In later years, dating multiple partners, and adolescent females dating older men are trouble indicators.

TROUBLE IN SCHOOL: Teens who get in trouble at school often engage in extreme behavior to gain attention from their peers.

USE OF ALCOHOL AND TOBACCO: Use of alcohol, tobacco or illegal drugs lowers inhibitions and can prompt throwing caution to the wind.

POOR GRADES IN SCHOOL: Troubled teens often seek alternative sources of excitement and achievement, and these alternatives include high risk sexual activity.

Although the early indicators listed above can help parents and other caring adults spot problems, teen pregnancy and sexually transmitted disease can also affect teens who do well, stay active in school, and abstain from harmful substances. It takes only one unprotected encounter to cause many problems.

Helping your teen develop a strong sense of self, high self-esteem, and a compelling belief in respectable values and ethical behavior, and encouraging him or her to set personal goals for the future are the best things you can do to prevent irresponsible sexual behavior.

EDUCATION IN SCHOOLS

Some parents do not feel they are competent enough to conduct conversations about sex. Still other parents are petrified that sex education will whet an appetite to experiment. However, education in the area of sexuality can be a cooperative venture between the family and schools. The overwhelming weight of evidence conducted by the National Campaign to Prevent Teen Pregnancy demonstrates that sexuality and HIV education, school-based clinics, and condom availability programs, do not increase any measure of sexual activity.

Initiatives in the schools, religious organizations, families and the community have had a pronounced impact on sexual behavior. Teenage birthrates nationwide declined substantially from 1991 to 1996, according to the National Center for Health Statistics. The sharpest declines were among black teenagers, until recently the group with the highest level of births. "What's significant is that these declines are in every state," says Donna E. Shalala, Secretary of Health and Human Services in 1999. "I give a lot of credit to the African-American community, which has put out a clear, consistent message from the churches, the schools and all sorts of civic organizations, a drumbeat to young women and young men that they should not become parents until they are truly ready to support a child, that having children too early will limit their options." Abstinence awareness programs

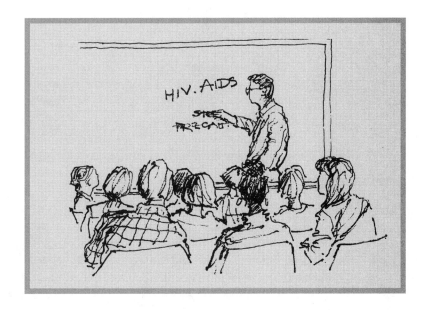

have been a contributing factor throughout the nation, but studies show that communities which embrace a wide assortment of education programs fare better than those which focus exclusively on abstinence. Check at your school to find out the types of programs offered to your teen.

MODELS OF PARENT-TEEN PROGRAMS

The National Campaign to Prevent Teen Pregnancy reports numerous success models of parent-teen-community awareness programs initiated across the country with federal aid to spark discussion. Here is a sampling: *Parents and Kids Learn Together* in St. Joseph, Missouri is an initiative using creative games to get parents and their children to talk and feel closer. In a *Dear Abby* game, groups of two parent-child couples are given a letter asking for advice about values, feelings, and beliefs related to sexuality, to which they must craft an answer together. The *Habla Con Tu Hermana (Talk with Your Sister)* program, which offers reproductive health advice and services to families in San Antonio, Texas, began in parents' homes but added outreach efforts. One component of the outreach includes two Spanish-speaking sisters who host an energetic call-in talk show on a wide variety of sexual and reproductive health issues. It sparks discussions about sex, values and relationships among parents and children. In New Orleans and Atlanta, parent led *Plain Talk Parties,* built on a party model, brings together small groups of parents in homes to discuss teen pregnancy and sexually-transmitted diseases, their impact on the community, and how adults can communicate effectively. Still other programs involve teens themselves creating newsletters, pamphlets and videos to alert each other about abstinence, safe sex and delayed gratification (See REFERENCES AND RESOURCES section).

SEXUAL ORIENTATION

Parents and caregivers who demonstrate by their own actions and teach their children to respect all individuals, do a service to all of humanity. Young people need support, not ridicule or shame, in coping with their lives today.

Sexual orientation, according to an article in the *Journal of Pediatric Health Care,* is believed to be influenced by a variety of factors, including genetics and hormones, as well as unknown environmental factors. The origins of sexual orientation are not understood and are controversial. The major point to keep in mind is that adolescents who are exploited, harassed, and rejected are at risk. This holds true for any adolescent. This risk includes risk of substance abuse, violence from others, and suicide. Fear and misinformation can be dispelled by careful review of materials found in the REFERENCES AND RESOURCES section at the end of the chapter on sexual harassment (Chapter 8). The philosophy advanced in this book is that all young people deserve to live in a world that is safe.

Sexually Transmitted Diseases (STDs)

The Case for Abstinence

If your teen does not have sex and does not inject drugs, you do not have to worry about him or her getting infected with sexually transmitted diseases (STDs).

"Abstinence is the only sure protection," says Dr. Mary L. Kamb, an epidemiologist at the Centers for Disease Control and Prevention (CDC).

Millions of teens do not have sexual intercourse. But 40 percent of ninth graders nationally and 66 percent of high school seniors do. Only 40 percent of teenagers seek contraceptive help in the first year of sexual activity, states Dr. Anita Nelson, Medical Director of the Women's Health Care clinic at Harbor University of California Medical Center, citing data from the Alan Guttmacher Institute.

> **Abstinence is the only sure protection.**

Health officials describe abstinence as "choosing not to engage in certain behaviors such as sexual intercourse or drug use." Abstinence means making a commitment and consistently avoiding certain behaviors—any time, any day, and under any circumstances. Parents and other concerned adults should talk to teens about the desirability of abstinence, but they should also explain how to reduce risks associated with sexual activity. Almost every teen will eventually become sexually active and have a need for such information, preferably as an adult.

To date, there is no known cure for the HIV infection. For many people, that fact alone is enough to make a case for abstinence to their teen. For other people, the facts about HIV and AIDS are only part of the larger picture that makes abstinence for their teen the right idea.

Obviously, your stance on abstinence is a personal one. No one wants to put his or her child at risk to life-threatening situations. Most people, however, still struggle with finding appropriate behaviors that allow teens to express intimacy, caring, and love. It is this gray area that adults and teens need to explore together—on the one hand, saying absolutely "no" to certain behaviors while, on the other hand, having normal feelings of caring and sharing. Your teen wants to hear from you how to grow and develop into an adult. Abstinence is an adult issue, and like many adult issues, it takes strength, caring, compassion, and discipline, often in equal measure and at nearly the same time. Working with your teen on abstinence and other adult issues is a powerful gift to give your teen.

The Human Immunodeficiency Virus (HIV)

As adolescent sexual activity has increased, so have rates of sexually transmitted diseases. The most deadly is HIV, which leads to the acquired immunodeficiency syndrome (AIDS). The CDC reports one-quarter of the estimated 40,000 new HIV infections in the United States probably occur in people under the age of 20 years. HIV is the seventh leading cause of death among people ages 15 to 24, according to Youth Risk Behavior Surveys (YRBS) analyzed by the CDC. Even though advances in medicine have helped curb the epidemic, it is far from over.

"Many teens infected with HIV show few symptoms because they are at the early stages of the disease," said *Straight Talk,* a magazine for teens. AIDS is the late stage of infection by HIV. Over time this virus severely weakens the immune system, resulting in AIDS. People might die from pneumonia and tuberculosis, for example, because their immune systems can no longer fight diseases or infections. Once infected, the best advice is to get tested and treated early.

Sandy Thurman, AIDS Policy Director to the U.S. President, has this to say: "AIDS is not curable. It can kill you. [If you can be treated], you'll have to take 30 pills a day, and the pills are like poison. If you're sexually active, safe sex is the ticket." Thurman begs people to tell their children AIDS is not a gay disease. "Fifty percent of new [U.S.] cases are related to drug use. One in four is a teen . . . We have to focus on the epidemic as it is today, not on how it was." Only a vaccine to prevent HIV can stop AIDS. She hopes for one by 2008. "It's a tall order. Even with polio, where there's been a cheap, easy vaccine for 40 years, we haven't eradicated it. If we don't find an HIV vaccine, hundreds of millions will die."

While HIV is the most deadly sexually transmitted disease (STD), teens can be infected with up to 25 different STDs. Every year, three million American teens contract an STD. One in four sexually active teens will contract an STD by the time they reach 21. Some STDs, such as gonorrhea, increase the risk of contracting HIV by creating skin lesions that make it easier to acquire the deadly virus. It is now recommended that all persons diagnosed with an STD be routinely tested for HIV.

> Fifty percent of new [U.S.] cases are related to drug use. One in four is a teen . . .
> — Sandy Thurman,
>   AIDS Policy Director
>   to the U.S. President

A front page *New York Times* article of August 31, 1999, reports that the rate of infection with the AIDS virus (HIV) is no longer declining in this country. And while the rate of AIDS deaths continues to fall, that rate of decline has slowed. The article continues to say that new infections with HIV were "dangerously high" in some areas among young gay men and heterosexual women, particularly blacks and members of other minorities. "In this era of better therapies, it is clear that people are becoming complacent about prevention," said Dr. Helene Gayle, who directs the AIDS program for the Centers for Disease Control and Prevention. "Nationwide, AIDS deaths dropped 42 percent from 1996 to 1997 but only 20 percent from 1997 to 1998. Although the death rates are much lower than they were at their peak in the 1980's, the slowing rate of decline shows that more aggressive prevention efforts are needed," Dr. Gayle said.

The Most Common STD's

CHLAMYDIA, a pelvic infection caused by the chlamydia trachomatis bacteria, is the fastest-spreading STD in the country. It is also the most reported STD in the U.S.

The infection is usually without symptoms, but if it is detected, it is easily treatable with antibiotics. Undetected, it can lead to the more serious pelvic inflammatory disease, and possible infertility (See symptom list on p. 84).

GONORRHEA ranks among the oldest and most contagious diseases. The infection is caused by the gonococcus bacteria, which incubates and multiplies in moist, warm areas of the body such as the cervix, urethra, mouth and rectum. It can be contracted by genital or oral sex with someone who is infected. If treated, it can be cured with antibiotics. Left untreated, the bacteria can spread to the bloodstream and infect the joints, heart valves or the brain. Like chlamydia, gonorrhea can also lead to pelvic inflammatory disease and infertility.

SYPHILIS is caused by treponema pallidum bacteria, which is spread through sores of an infected person. While new cases of the disease have fallen to their lowest rates in 40 years, left untreated it spreads to the bones, spinal chord and the heart. It can cause insanity and death. Treatment with antibiotics can cure the disease.

GENITAL HERPES is incurable and is usually caused by sexual contact with someone who has an outbreak of herpes sores in the genital area. The herpes simplex virus comes in two forms. Type 1 usually causes sores on the lips; type 2 most often causes genital sores. An estimated 40 million Americans have herpes, a disease which returns with outbreaks on regular intervals. Untreated pregnant women with herpes often transmit it to their babies during childbirth. In babies, herpes can be fatal.

HEPATITIS B is transmitted by direct contact with the blood or body fluids of an infected person. Hepatitis B spreads through sexual intercourse, unsanitized needles applied through steroid injections, body piercing and tattooing. A hepatitis B vaccine is available at most doctors' offices and public health clinics, which will prevent a person from getting this disease.

THE HUMAN PAPILLOMA VIRUS (HPV) infects as many as one million Americans each year in more than 70 different types. The disease ranges from harmless warts on the hands or feet to genital warts, which can lead to cervical cancer in women. A person can have an HPV infection without warts or other symptoms. Genital warts can be removed through medication applied directly to the warts, drug therapy or surgery. Several treatments might be needed to clear genital warts, and treatment does not always kill all infected cells. Genital warts is not curable.

Sexually Transmitted Diseases (STDs): The Facts

The *Weekly Reader Current Health 2® Magazine* suggests that parents, caregivers, and teens review the facts about sexually transmitted diseases (STDs), including HIV infection and chlamydia. Here are a few pointers. These facts apply to all STDs:

- You cannot tell by looking at someone whether he or she is infected with an STD.

- There are often no symptoms early in an infection. When symptoms do occur, they are often confused with other illnesses.
- The more partners a person has, the higher the chance of being exposed to HIV and other STDs.
- Using drugs and alcohol increases the risk of getting STDs because they lower inhibitions. Under the influence of such substances, people often do not use a condom properly or remember the next day what they did the night before.
- Intravenous drug use puts a person at higher risk for HIV and hepatitis B, because IV drug users often share needles.

Special permission granted, *Current Health 2 Magazine*, ©1998 published by Weekly Reader Corporation. All rights reserved.

Symptoms that Might Indicate a Sexually Transmitted Disease (STD):

- Discharge from the vagina, penis, or rectum.
- Pain or burning during urination or intercourse.
- Pain in the abdomen (women), testicles (men), or buttocks and legs (both).
- Blisters, open sores, warts, rash, or swelling in the genital or anal areas, lips, mouth, or throat.
- Persistent flu-like symptoms, including fever, headache, aching muscles, or swollen glands.

Special permission granted, *Current Health 2® Magazine*, ©1998 published by Weekly Reader Corporation. All rights reserved.

It is important to remember that many people have STDs without any obvious signs. If a person thinks they are at risk they should seek medical help. People who are sexually active with a new partner, with multiple partners, or with a partner who has multiple partners or injects drugs, should get tested by a physician or at a health clinic regularly, to protect themselves and their partner from STDs. Immediate attention to symptoms is important. Proper use of a latex condom is the best protection against the spread of disease, but additional use of spermicides and diaphragms could be helpful. Remember that latex condoms are the only contraceptive labeled by the Food and Drug Administration to be effective in preventing sexual transmission of HIV.

Piercing, Tattooing and Needle Sharing

The youth culture thrives on adopting new, outrageous styles that infuriate parents and bond youth with one another. Two of the newer, more dangerous trends include body piercing and tattooing. In fact, the American Dental Association passed a resolution in 1996 to oppose oral piercing, which it considers a public health hazard. Enthusiasts pay friends and unlicensed practitioners $50 or more to punch a hole through their lips, cheek or tongue with mouth jewelry. Some of the piercing is done at parties where needles are shared and unsanitized.

Whenever unsanitized needles are involved, the blood from one person is injected into another. If that blood is infected it could carry hepatitis B, HIV and other diseases. Foreign material, ink or jewelry compound the risk. For that reason, blood donations cannot be made for a year after getting a tattoo, body piercing, or permanent makeup.

The risk is equally great for tattooing, which could lead to infectious diseases or permanent skin discoloration. Tattoos are open wounds that can become infected. The new tattoo must be kept clean and must be kept moist with an ointment to prevent a scab from forming.

Yet another risk comes from injecting steroids to increase muscle mass for improved sports performance. The Olympics disqualify anyone found to use drugs to improve athletic performance. But some youth want to achieve prized honors that could lead to glory and scholarship. Steroids are notoriously unstable and unsanitized needles carry the same risk as seen for piercing or tattooing.

> Whenever unsanitized needles are involved, the blood from one person is injected into another. If that blood is infected it could carry hepatitis B, HIV and other diseases.

References & Resources   R/R

Author's Note: Parents, caregivers and educators might want to read these materials to evaluate suitability for their adolescent or students.

Sexual Issues

The 500 Year Delta: What Happens After What Comes Next, Jim Taylor and Watts Wacker (Harper Business, 1998, $14.00). These futurists talk about a number of trends including youth lifestyles and interests, including androgyny, the growing similarity in clothing styles and haircuts between males and females.

"The Bully in the Mirror", Stephen S. Hall, in *The New York Times Magazine,* August 22, 1999. This article describes how cultural messages about an ideal male body have grown more insistent, more aggressive, more widespread and more explicit in recent years, and the effects this is having on boys.

Daughters (Pleasant Company Publications, 8400 Fairway Place, Middleton WI 53562, one year/eight issues for $39.95). *Daughters* is an outstanding, nationally acclaimed newsletter written to help build strong parent-daughter relationships.

How to Talk with Your Teenagers About the Facts of Life, Planned Parenthood Federation of America, Inc. (Marketing Department, 810 7th Ave., New York, NY 10010, 800-669-0156 or a local office, 1999, $3.00). Straight answers to most-asked questions about puberty, reproduction, pregnancy, contraception, and sexuality.

My Body, My Self, Lynda Madaras and Area Madaras (Newmarket Press, 1995, $11.95). Illustrations, quizzes, and exercises for preteen and teenage girls exploring the physical changes of puberty.

Parenting Solutions, Manisses Communications Group, Inc., (P.O. Box 9758, Providence, RI 02940-9758). Provides teen-oriented flyers on a variety of parenting topics, including sex education.

Sexuality Information and Education Council of the United States (SIECUS). (212-819-9770, 130 West 42nd Street, Suite 35, New York NY 10036). Provides information on sexuality for educators and parents. Offers *SIECUS Report,* (Sex Information & Educational, April/May 1993, $9.20). In a society where less than 10 percent of today's young people receive comprehensive sex education, the SIECUS guidelines offer comprehensive guidelines for grades K-12. Offers *Facing Facts: Sexual Health for America's Adolescents* (The Report of the National Commission on Adolescent Sexual Health), written in plain language. Web site: www.siecus.org.

Talking About Sex: A Guide for Families. Planned Parenthood Federation of America, (800-829-7732, 810 Seventh Avenue, New York, NY 10019, $29.95). On-line ordering available for this video and many other materials. Much information provided free on this extensive Web site, available in English and Spanish. Call 800-669-0156 for ordering. A video kit, with parent's guide and children's activity workbook, designed to help kids and parents get through puberty. A thoughtful and entertaining video that will provide parents with the knowledge and role modeling to help them be more comfortable talking to their kids about sexuality (see Planned Parenthood listing). Web site: www.plannedparenthood.org.

Talking With Your Teen About Sex and *Talking With Your Child About Sex.* These pamphlets can be accessed at the National Parent-Teacher's Association (PTA) Web site. The version for parents of teens addresses HIV/AIDS, peer pressure avoidance skills, and date rape. The second pamphlet offers information about reproduction, the importance of strengthening self-esteem in the early years, and the necessity of communicating values. The Web site offers an extensive set of archives of pamphlets, publications, reports, handbooks, photographs, etc on a wide variety of subjects. Web site: www.pta.org (to get directly to the archives, go to www.pta.org/apta/archrs.htm.)

Talking to Your Young Teen About Sex and Sexuality: Guidelines for Parents, American Academy of Pediatrics Division of Publications, (141 Northwest Point Blvd, PO Box 927, Elk Grove Village IL 60009-01997, 1997, minimum order 100 @ $24.95 per 100). A sample of the contents of this pamphlet can be found within this chapter.

Transitions (Advocates for Youth, Suite 200, 1025 Vermont Avenue NW, Washington DC 20005,
202-347-5700, 202-347-2263-fax. E-mail address: info@advocatesforyouth.org. Web site:
www.advocatesforyouth.org., one year subscription $28.00) *Transitions* is a quarterly
publication of Advocates for Youth—helping young people make safe and responsible decisions
about sex. In June 1999, Advocates for Youth announced the opening of The Center for Adolescent
Health & the Law (A Project of Advocates for Youth, 211 North Columbia Street, Chapel
Hill NC 27514, 919-968-8850, 919-968-8854-fax. E-mail address: info@adolescenthealthlaw.org.
Web site: www.adolescenthealthlaw.org). The Center will provide critical research to inform
the public policy debate on issues affecting young people's health, including their sexual and
reproductive health. The Center will conduct research, analyze legal and policy issues, prepare
publications, provide training and technical assistance, and engage in advocacy.

The What's Happening to My Body Book for Girls, and *The What's Happening to My Body Book for Boys,*
Lynda Madaras (Newmarket Press, 1995, $11.95) Written for parents and their daughters
and sons, this is a guide to the changes of puberty, along with information on AIDS, sexually
transmitted disease, and birth control.

Pregnancy Prevention

Considering Your Options: Information on Abstinence and Contraceptive Choices for Teenagers. Video. National
Education Association Health Information Network. (NEA Professional Library Distribution
Center, PO Box 2035, Annapolis Junction MD 20701-2035, 800-229-4200, 301-206-9789-fax,
$15.00). This is a fast-paced video that combines animated segments where a teen goes on-line
to learn more about contraceptive options and segments where real teens discuss their choices
and concerns about sexual activity and various birth control methods.

Heat of the Moment. Video (Mississippi Department of Human Services, PO Box 352, 750 North State St,
Jackson MS 39205, $10.00). This 18-minute video features teens telling their actual stories about
their problems and decisions. This unscripted documentary brings the viewer face to face with
the innermost struggles of teens. Their lives, their thoughts and their day-to-day hardships are
openly revealed as they deal with the consequences of having sex or their decision to just wait.

The Kaiser Family Foundation. (2400 Sand Hill Rd., Menlo Park, CA, 94025, 650-854-9400). Provides a variety
of resources about teen pregnancy; they also conduct research on adolescent sex issues.
Web site: www.kff.org/homepage.

The National Campaign to Prevent Teen Pregnancy, (2100 M Street NW, Suite 300, Washington, DC 20037,
202-261-5655, 202-331-7735-fax). The National Campaign is a nonprofit, nonpartisan initiative
supported almost entirely by private donations. The Campaign's strategy involves working with
the entertainment media, parents, and others to change the teen culture, and working with local
communities to build a more coordinated and effective grassroots movement. Both components
are anchored in strong research on effective approaches and respect for the role of religion and
values in shaping solutions. They publish a series of brochures about national efforts underway
to reduce adolescent birth rates. Among their publications are *Ten Tips for Parents to Help Their
Children Avoid Teen Pregnancy,* and *Nine Tips to Help Faith Leaders and Their Communities
Address Teen Pregnancy.* An extensive set of resources are available on-line at their Web site,
with on-line ordering for brochures, pamphlets, etc. Or order by fax at above fax number.
Up to 10 copies of each publication is free of charge. Web site: www.teenpregnancy.org.

A Parent Handbook for Talking with Adolescents About Sex and Birth Control, J. Jaccard and P. Dittus
(Department of Psychology, University at Albany, State University of New York, Albany NY 12222,
1999, 518-442-4864, 518-442-4867-fax. E-mail address: jjj20@csc.albany.edu.). This manual, which
is the culmination of over 20 years of research on this topic by Dr. Jaccard, will be available
as of March 2000.

Partners in Prevention: How National Organizations Assist State and Local Teen Pregnancy Prevention Efforts
(National Campaign to Prevent Teen Pregnancy, 1997, $18.00). For order information, see National
Campaign listing above. Based on a survey of 80 national organizations, this guide describes the

kinds of assistance and resources each national group offers state and local teen pregnancy prevention efforts.

Planned Parenthood Federation of America: 800-829-7732 (810 Seventh Avenue, New York, NY 10019). The mission of Planned Parenthood is: to provide comprehensive reproductive and complementary health care services in settings which preserve and protect the essential privacy and rights of each individual; to advocate public policies which guarantee these rights and ensure access to such services; to provide educational programs which enhance understanding of individual and societal implications of human sexuality; to promote research and the advancement of technology in reproductive health care and encourage understanding of their inherent bioethical, behavioral, and social implications. E-mail address: communications@ppfa.org. Web site: www.plannedparenthood.org.

Power In Numbers: Peer Effects on Adolescent Girls' Sexual Debut and Pregnancy, Peter Bearman and Hannah Brückner (The National Campaign to Prevent Teen Pregnancy, 1999). When it comes to the influence teens have on each other, many parents and other adults fear the worst. They not only believe that peers are the major influence on the decisions adolescents make about sex and other matters, but they also believe that peer influence is invariably negative. This document presents an in-depth research-based analysis exploring some of these assumptions about peer influence, with surprising findings. This information is also available in a condensed version entitled *Peer Potential: Making the Most of How Teens Influence Each Other.* See National Campaign listing above for ordering information.

ReCAPP (Resource Center for Adolescent Pregnancy Prevention) is a Web site that provides practical tools and information on reducing sexual risk-taking behaviors among teens. It has information on evidence-based programs and effective practices that change sexual risk-taking behavior; abstracts, news summaries and the latest statistics on teen pregnancy; and a resource database of educational materials. Web site: www.etr.org/recapp.

Sex Smart: 501 Reasons to Hold Off on Sex, Susan Browning Pogany (Fairview Press, 1998, $14.95). This is an abstinence resource for teens. It addresses teens in an honest and conversational style, making a strong case for sexual responsibility. The book features teens and their stories about abstinence and about sexual experiences.

Snapshots from the Front Line: Lessons About Teen Pregnancy Prevention from States and Communities, 1997. *Snapshots from the Front Line II: Lessons from Programs that Involve Parents and Other Adults in Preventing Teen Pregnancy,* 1998. (The National Campaign to Prevent Teen Pregnancy, Washington DC. For ordering information, see National Campaign listing above. One copy free, additional copies $5.00). The National Campaign has paid visits to programs across the nation to catalyze and support efforts in pregnancy prevention. The booklets are not only inspirational but can be of real help, as can the organization, in assisting communities and states. *Snapshots II* contains telephone contacts for the programs featured.

Talking Back: Ten Things Teens Want Parents to Know About Teen Pregnancy (National Campaign to Prevent Teen Pregnancy, 1999, up to five copies free. For ordering information, see National Campaign listing above). This offers answers to the question: If you could give your parents and other important adults advice about how to help you and your friends avoid pregnancy, what would it be?

Thinking About the Right-Now: What Teens Want Other Teens to Know About Preventing Pregnancy (National Campaign to Prevent Teen Pregnancy, 1999, up to five copies free. For ordering information, see National Campaign listing above). This advice—for teens, from teens—is based on suggestions offered by readers of *Teen People* magazine, the Campaign's own Youth Leadership Team, and teen visitors to the Campaign's Web site.

"We Care...We Act," The American Association of School Administrators (Direct inquires to Sharon Adams-Taylor, Director of Children's Initiatives, AASA, 1801 North Moore Street, Arlington, VA 22209). Brochure about teenage pregnancy prevention and other sex topics, which details what it takes to support and nurture healthy teen growth and development. Web site: www.aasa.org/issues/advocacy/wecare_act.htm.

Sexually Transmitted Diseases (STDs)

Advocates for Youth, 202-347-5700. (1025 Vermont Ave NW Suite 210, Washington DC 20005).
  Offers resources for teachers on how to develop educational programs wherein young people
  counsel one another on HIV. Has a quarterly newsletter, *Transitions,* designed to keep teachers,
  counselors, and other professionals up to date on adolescent health and sexuality issues.

AIDS-Proofing Your Kids: A Step-by-Step Guide, Loren Acker, Bram Gold-water, William Dyson (Beyond Words
  Publishing Co., 1992, $8.95). Stresses parental involvement in educating teenagers about AIDS
  with a collection of practical, direct, and easily understood strategies for approaching the topic
  comfortably and effectively.

Centers for Disease Control (CDC) National Hot Lines. For more information or to speak to someone about
  sexually transmitted diseases:
      CDC National AIDS Hotline: 800-342-2437-English, 800-344-7432-Spanish
      CDC National AIDS Clearinghouse: 800-458-5231. Web site: www.cdcnac.org.
      CDC National STD Hotline: 800-227-8922.

Clinical Trials: 800-TRIALS-A (800-874-2572). Source of the National Institutes of Allergy and Infectious
  Diseases. Offers latest on all AIDS studies.

Current Health 2® Magazine, with Human Sexuality Supplement. (Contact: Subscriber Services, 800-446-3355.
  Current Health 2, Weekly Reader Corp., 3001 Cindel Drive, Delron NJ 08370). *Current Health 2*
  magazine covers a range of topics from STDs to teen hormones, and is published eight times
  during the school year. Volume 24, No. 6, February 1998 provides extensive STD information.
  Web site: www.weeklyreader.com.

Deciding About Sex: The Choice to Abstain (#138) and *STD Facts* (#153, or #165 in Spanish). Network
  Publications (P.O. Box 1830, Santa Cruz, CA 95061-1830. Call 800-321-4407 for free catalog
  and pamphlets).

Herpes Resource Center: 800-230-6039. Web site: http://sunsite.unc.edu/ ASHA/.

How to Protect Yourself from AIDS. Contact for free copies of pamphlets: U.S. Department of Health
  and Human Services, Food and Drug Administration, Communications Staff (HFI-40),
  Rockville, MD 20857.

*Michigan Sex Education and HIV/STD Prevention Program Guide: A Guide to Selecting Effective Pregnancy
  Prevention, HIV Prevention, and STD Prevention Programs and Strategies for Grades 7-12.* (Michigan
  Department of Education, 517-373-7247). This guide was developed by the Michigan Department
  of Education in partnership with the Michigan Department of Community Health, to provide
  information that will assist Michigan schools and community organizations in selecting resources
  for middle school and high school students. It provides a wealth of information about the content
  and evaluation of 15 secondary programs, including both abstinence-based and abstinence-only
  alternatives. The guide may be copied and distributed, as it was developed with public funds.

The National AIDS Hotline: 800-342-AIDS-English, 800-344-7432-Spanish, 800-243-7889-TDD. Provides
  referrals to local AIDS organizations as well as general information and education.

National AIDS Hotline for Teenagers. 800-234-8336. Offers young people information, counseling,
  and support.

Straight Talk: A Magazine for Teens, (Learning Partnership, Inc., PO Box 199, Pleasantville, NY 10570-0199,
  914-769-0055). Published periodically for teenagers, *Straight Talk* offers an excellent series
  of teen-oriented publications about STDs, relationships and substance abuse.

Teen Choices: 817-237-0230-phone, 817-238-2048-fax. Provides HIV/STD education programs
  to schools and churches. Develops and distributes HIV/STD education materials.
  E-mail address: teenchoice@aol.com.

What Parents Need to Tell Children About AIDS (1992). *A Close Encounter* (1988). *Flirting With Danger*
  (1994), New York State Department of Health (Health Education Services, A Division of Health
  Research Inc., P.O. Box 7126, Albany, NY 12224, 518-439-7286). These publications can be
  purchased for 75¢ each. Catalog available. The last two publications are in full-color, comic

book format. Easy-to-read, but contain explicit graphics and subject matter with story lines on avoiding AIDS.

Tattooing/Piercing

Prevention Researcher Newsletter, Integrated Research Services, Inc. (66 Club Road, Suite 370, Eugene, Oregon, 97401-2464, 800-929-2955). This newsletter is published tri-annually by Integrated Research Services, a non-profit research and educational corporation specializing in substance abuse prevention and human performance. For specific information on health risks of tattooing and piercing, from educators and prevention personnel affiliated with the newsletter, please see volume 5, No.3. Web site: www.integres.org/prevres/.

CHAPTER 5
TEENS: AN ACTIVE LIFESTYLE

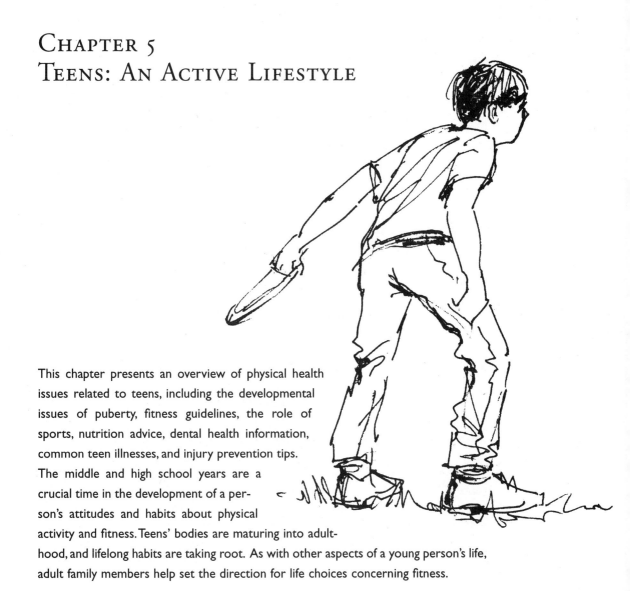

This chapter presents an overview of physical health issues related to teens, including the developmental issues of puberty, fitness guidelines, the role of sports, nutrition advice, dental health information, common teen illnesses, and injury prevention tips. The middle and high school years are a crucial time in the development of a person's attitudes and habits about physical activity and fitness. Teens' bodies are maturing into adulthood, and lifelong habits are taking root. As with other aspects of a young person's life, adult family members help set the direction for life choices concerning fitness.

PUBERTY: THE GREAT DIVIDE

Emotional Development

The title of this section and inspiration for its writing draws from the 1995 *Your Child's Emotional Health* by Jack Maguire, with deep thanks for the sensitive writing found in the book. *Your Child's Emotional Health* comes from the work of the medical staff of the Philadelphia Guidance Center, one of the foremost centers in the country for child and adolescent psychiatric care. A second very readable and useful introductory resource on the physical development of young women and young men during puberty comes from pediatrician and educator Chrystal de Freitas' *Keys to Your Child's Healthy Sexuality.*

A quote from *Your Child's Emotional Health* reinforces the overall philosophy of *Healthy Teens*—that of helping adults understand both the emotional and physical development of their child. The author states, "...the dividing line between childhood and adolescence is puberty. Regardless of a child's specific age, grade in school, personal responsibilities, or degree of social maturity, she or he cannot be considered an adult (or, more precisely, a person becoming an adult) until puberty has begun working its hormonal revolution in all aspects of the child's life. Parents of teenage children need to be particularly sensitive to their child's needs during this major transitional period in her or his development, for the very beginning of adulthood often determines how the eventual adult will turn out—not just physically, but also emotionally."

Text in *Your Child's Emotional Health* reminds adults that it is a good idea to celebrate your child's entry into puberty with a special occasion—a special gift or ceremony. You and your pre-adolescent can decide on when that entry into adulthood is occurring. The discussion of physical changes that follow may be helpful.

Moreover, the book recommends skipping humor and teasing responses to the changes in your young person (there will be enough of that from friends and uninformed adults.) Help your youngster believe that during this period of physical changes and the accompanying emotional stress that change brings, adulthood is a new, wonderful time in one's life. The authors say, "Present it (puberty) as a desirable and positive stage of growth—linked with beauty, power, and a rich new range of feelings."

Other authorities explain that most parents are aware of the turmoil adolescence can bring; they remember their own adolescent years with mixed feelings. Some may be saddened as their child begins to separate from them, while still others may welcome the intellectual growth of their teen. Many worry about potential risky behavior. Events of the present can combine with an adult's recollections of their past and the process of their own adolescence, as they strive to support their teen through this process.

It is wise to be reminded that, while a daughter's waistline becomes more pronounced or a son looks like he needs to shave, they are not necessarily adults. It takes time to be responsible, behave thoughtfully, and have empathy for the world's social problems. A helpful guideline to use is to allow your child to mature mentally, socially, and emotionally during puberty at the same pace as he or she did before puberty.

During puberty, parents and caregivers will encounter mood swings in their children. Physicians believe the mood swings are related to hormonal changes during puberty. This is not the time to allow free wheeling back talk and get involved in shouting matches. Mood swings are not an excuse for rudeness and disrespect toward anyone. As always, the adults need to take the lead in being mature and correct foul language and inappropriate behavior. In addition, it takes considerable patience to find a way to spend time with a child whose mood seems to change every twenty minutes. Let your youngster know how much you love him or her and try to find a mutual ground so you can spend some time together. Remember, mood swings are upsetting to your emerging adolescent, too. You need to be there to give reassurance that moods can be helped with quiet time, exercise, breathing exercises, and other forms of relaxation. You need to keep connected; your moral guidance is vitally important.

While institutions in society help young people to learn, to choose how they will worship, to serve others, to find entertainment and friends, and to prepare for further study and work, it is the family that provides the bedrock foundation of love, support, and moral guidance that makes puberty successful. This includes helping teens understand they need to be responsible for their emerging sexual urges.

PHYSICAL DEVELOPMENT: YOUR DAUGHTER IN PUBERTY

For most girls, puberty begins around age nine or ten, although it may start anytime from age eight to fifteen years. If a young woman is fifteen years old and has not experienced any of the sexual changes associated with puberty, she should see a physician. Puberty in girls can take from one-and-a-half years to five years, with an average of four years.

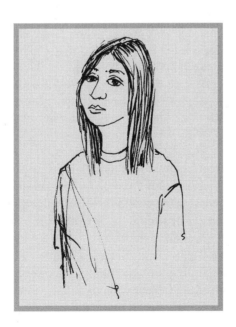

A young daughter usually has some breast development and pubic hair before her first period, but adult breast size and mature pubic hair distribution will not be completed until some time later. If a girl has her first period before any breast development, she should visit a physician to make sure there is no underlying physical disorder. The sequence during your daughter's puberty occurs in the following order: breast buds; growth spurt; pubic hair; first menstruation (menarche); underarm hair; and growth of uterus and vagina completed.

The development of breasts is one of the earliest signs of puberty in about eighty-five percent of girls. Most girls develop breasts between the ages of eight and thirteen. The progression of breast development is gradual. It can take four to five years to complete. Some girls, though, grow more quickly and reach maturity in one or two years. There is no way to speed up growth or, for that matter, to slow it down. Young girls may notice some small lumpiness underneath the nipple area in the very early stages of breast development. This area may feel tender, but it is, in fact, normal. Glandular tissue that will later contribute to the production of breast milk for nursing a baby is located there. It is also not unusual for one breast to grow larger than the other. This initial unevenness is common, and eventually both breasts usually grow to about the same size.

Some pre-adolescents worry about what the size of their breasts will be once fully developed. It is important to reassure your daughter that she will develop the breasts that are just the right size for her. Nothing that she does, or does not do, will influence the natural appearance of her breasts. Breast development is predetermined by genes, the same as height and eye color. Society's emphasis on breast size as an attractive aspect of femininity is an unfortunate reality. However, breast size has no impact on your daughter's ability to produce breast milk or her ability to have a satisfying sexual life.

When a young girl begins to notice her nipples protruding, or her breasts becoming tender, she might want to wear a piece of clothing between her chest and the outer layer. A camisole, training bra, sports bra, or undervest are choices. Girls may be uncomfortable asking about how to deal with developing breasts, so adults may have to take the initiative and suggest the next step. Some girls are very sensitive about the idea of wearing a bra, though there are those at the other end of the spectrum who cannot wait to wear one.

Fathers who are raising daughters by themselves may want to call upon their sister or a female friend to help their daughter at this time. If questions about physical development and sexuality have been addressed sensitively throughout childhood, fathers can feel secure in helping during this developmental time.

Most girls experience the beginning of their growth spurt around age nine, but a rapid spurt can start as late as thirteen. The greatest increase in height occurs early in puberty, with only limited growth after menarche. In young women, curves around the hips become more pronounced as fat accumulates in response to hormonal changes. The waist becomes more defined, and new body contours define a changing shape. During puberty's growth spurt, ninety-five percent of girls gain between twelve and twenty-three pounds per year. Once a girl starts menstruating, her growth and weight gain slow down, and she reaches her final adult height approximately two years later.

Adults may notice their pre-teen's body odor as early as seven or eight years of age. Usually, these youngsters are not aware of this odor, and they may be insulted when it is pointed out to them. Nevertheless, a gentle reminder about the need to take regular showers and to use deodorant or antiperspirants is necessary.

Shortly after the development of breasts in girls, hair will appear in new places on the body: legs, armpits, and in the pubic area. Hair growth is a gradual process and usually goes unnoticed. Underarm hair usually develops between the ages of twelve and thirteen in girls. In some cultures, females do not shave their underarm hair, but, in others, it is more customary to do so. Whether or not to shave is a personal choice.

Menstruation

Menstruation is an important event in the life of a young girl. It marks her passage into womanhood. Adults can make their daughters feel comfortable with this natural, monthly function by introducing the topic of menstruation early and often enough that their youngster's questions are completely addressed and any fears they have are allayed, long before the event occurs. It is the suddenness of menstruation that frightens an unprepared early teen.

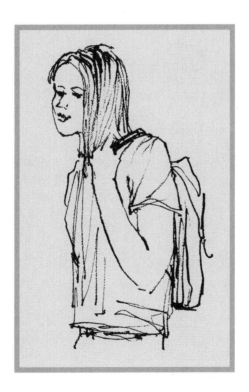

If a daughter is eight or nine years old and you have not discussed male and female body parts, intercourse, and how pregnancy occurs, this discussion needs to happen prior to explaining menstruation. Following that understanding, here are the simple facts:

- Menstruation is the way the female body prepares for a possible pregnancy.
- Menstruation happens to all girls when they start puberty.
- Menstruation is a very natural and normal part of growing up.

The first menstrual cycle (menarche) can occur anytime from age nine until as late as sixteen. It usually occurs about two years after breast budding. Menstruation is also referred to as "having your period." Be careful to explain this process well. Most women long remember the explanation and their first period.

As Dr. deFreitas indicates, "Menstruation is regulated by a gland in the brain called the pituitary gland. The pituitary gland acts as an internal clock that awakens and signals the beginning of puberty at precisely the right time for each person. . . Hormones are substances. . . that are responsible for the changes associated with puberty. . . The ovaries are the female's sex organs. They produce one of the body's hormones, estrogen, and they store a woman's egg cells (ova). A woman is born with a fixed number of egg cells, 400,000 to be exact. . . Triggered by the body's hormones, these ova begin to mature and are released from the ovaries. This process is called ovulation. Although several egg cells can mature at a time, usually only one ovum is released from the ovary during each menstrual cycle. At the same time, the uterus prepares for the possibility of pregnancy."

When the ovum is released, it travels along the fallopian tube. If the ovum is not fertilized, it travels toward the uterus during the next several days. Two weeks after ovulation, the dissolved ovum, along with the lining of the uterus, is shed. This lining, consisting of blood-tinged fluid, constitutes the menstrual flow.

The menstrual flow leaves the body through the vagina, the opening between the woman's legs that is also the birth canal. The menstrual flow can last from two days to as many as seven, with an average of three to five days. The flow is a slow, steady trickle, as opposed to a sudden gush of fluid, and the body easily replaces the lost blood. It is normal for the menstrual flow to sometimes contain blood clots and small pieces of tissue.

The menstrual cycle is counted from the first day of the menstrual flow to the first day of the next one. Menstruation occurs approximately every twenty-eight to forty days, or on the average, once a month. It is common for menstrual cycles to be irregular for the first year or two, and some girls may skip several months in a row or have a period every two weeks.

Some girls may not get their periods until they are in high school, and that is perfectly fine. Just because a teen is fourteen and she has not gotten her period yet does not necessarily mean that anything is wrong with her. Some young women, though, may not be getting their first periods because of other reasons:

- Some girls who are very athletic may not get their period until they stop exercising or competing so vigorously.
- Girls who are underweight or overweight may notice a delay in the beginning of their period.
- Just like stress can lead to tense back muscles, it can also delay menstruation.
- Having certain illnesses may interfere with the start of periods.
- Remember that it is possible for a girl to get pregnant before she gets her first period. Being pregnant would mean that she would not get her period.

Physical Development: Your Son in Puberty

Most young men start their pubertal changes at age eleven or twelve. Male puberty can begin as early as age nine and as late as age fourteen. Changes occur over an average of three years, but can range from two to five years. Some males continue to grow into their late teens; this is normal.

Boys do not begin a growth spurt until after their sex organs begin to develop. Boys may grow about three to five inches a year during their growth spurt. For most boys, this rapid growth occurs between twelve and fifteen years of age, and lasts for two to three years. Their bodies lose fat during puberty and muscle mass increases, particularly around their shoulders, arms, and thighs.

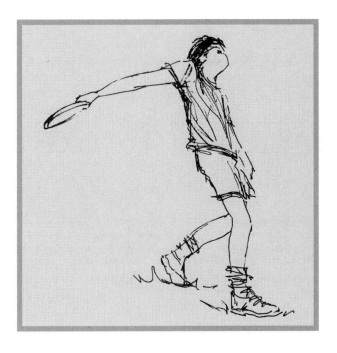

If your son has excessive acne at age ten, but no other physical characteristics of puberty, he should be evaluated by his physician. During puberty lumpiness might occur in your son's nipple area; this is normal. If this is upsetting to the teen, or if breast enlargement is pronounced, a physician should be consulted. If you son reaches fifteen, and shows no signs related to puberty, caring adults will want to see that a physician is consulted. A sensitive doctor who is good at communicating with teens and is trained in adolescent medicine can be located. Check with your own physician, friends, and a teaching or research hospital. See the REFERENCES AND RESOURCES section for a listing for the Society for Adolescent Medicine, which can provide information to help you locate a specialist in the field of adolescent medicine.

Most of the pubertal changes in boys overlap each other; therefore, several may occur at the same time. The general order of development of boys during puberty is as follows: growth of scrotum and testes; growth of penis; growth spurt; pubic hair; first ejaculation; voice change; and underarm hair. It will be very helpful to your son if you provide a carefully selected reference or two that describes the normal development of male sex characteristics. (See REFERENCES AND RESOURCES for a variety of sources.)

In general, during the first developmental stage in your son's puberty, the testes and scrotum enlarge and the skin of the scrotum may get darker. This is followed by the growth of the penis, and continued enlargement of the testicles and

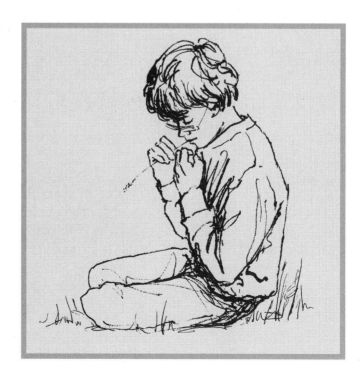

growth of pubic hair. At this time, one testicle may hang a bit lower than the other (this happens to prevent crushing against each other when males walk). When the adult stage has been reached, the penis is fully grown and the testes have reached full size, with one hanging somewhat lower than the other. Reassurance that each male's timetable of development is different is an important role for parents and caregivers. The size of the penis worries young men and assurances about this can be handled sensitively.

Beginning at puberty, boys' testes produce millions of spermatozoa, the male sex cells. A sperm is a microscopic cell shaped like a tadpole, which is carried in a clear or milky-colored fluid called semen. The semen leaves the body through the urethra, as does urine, but they never go through at the same time.

Erections

During puberty, an erection occurs as blood rushes to the penis; the penis gets hard and stands out. It may produce a bulge in the crotch area. Your son cannot always control whether or not he will have an erection, and during the early stages of puberty, spontaneous erections are very common. Furthermore, erections are not necessarily associated with sexual thoughts. The unpredictability of erections can be the most embarrassing and awkward aspect of puberty for boys. Reassure your sons that, for the most part, an erection is noticeable only to them. Help them figure out different ways to deal with an unpredictable erection: remain seated, cross or uncross legs, or hold a book in front of themselves. The erection goes away quickly. It is not necessary to have an ejaculation in order to end an erection, but often ejaculation occurs along with an orgasm. An orgasm is a series of contractions centered in the genital area. During an orgasm, the penis experiences a series of contractions that help spurt out the semen; it then becomes soft again. Ejaculations will begin about one year after penis growth begins—usually between ages twelve and fourteen.

Wet Dreams

Once the male body starts producing sperm, a boy may experience his first nocturnal emission, also known as a wet dream. This is an involuntary ejaculation that occurs only during sleep and is not necessarily associated with sexual thoughts. Most boys do experience wet dreams and they are entirely normal. Experiencing wet dreams can be confusing if you have not prepared your son. According to Dr. deFritas, the most common misinterpretation of this entirely normal event is that your son has wet his bed, or worse, that something is terribly wrong with him.

She also says that, as parents and caregivers, you can make sure that your son's accumulation of knowledge is accurate and is not grounded in myths. It is normal for him to be fascinated by the changes in his body. He need not feel frightened by them. Provide support and information, books he can read in private, and the reassurances he needs to be comfortable with his development.

HEALTH EDUCATION: LESSONS IN ADOLESCENT DEVELOPMENT

Some health education curricula offer fifth and sixth graders lessons in the basic physical and emotional changes of adolescence. One such curriculum is *Health 'n Me* (see REFERENCES AND RESOURCES). Review of health lesson materials by adults in the community is welcomed by school principals and teachers. Volunteering to serve on the district or local school health committee is one way to serve that purpose. Adults who believe that a health education program is important and want to facilitate its development in schools for all youngsters find the local or district health committee an important way to serve the community. These curriculum lessons related to puberty can be very helpful to families. It is important, however, that they are offered by a teacher with special training in adolescent development, that they are accompanied by suitable helpful information written by adolescent authorities, and that they are given ample opportunity for parental review and involvement. Usually, families welcome the assistance of the school as they carry on their own teaching related to adolescent development.

BUILDING AN ACTIVE LIFESTYLE

The family can have a powerful influence in directing their teen toward a healthy lifestyle by giving the proper messages, both by example and by encouragement. Teens need to learn that physical activity is important now, and throughout their lifetimes.

Little physical movement is involved in many of the activities of modern life, like sitting at a desk or computer, driving in a car, playing video games, or watching TV. Therefore, caring adults need to emphasize that physical activity must be sought out consciously. Adults need to set a clear, healthy example.

"The important message to get across to your teens," says Dr. David Rosen, Director of Teenage and Young Adult Health at the University of Michigan Medical Center, "is that physical activity does not need to be 'exercise'. The old concept of forty minutes of exercise that raises your heart rate is outmoded. Any amount of activity will add up to improving health—walking, going upstairs, mowing the lawn."

Physical Activity and Health

Though the importance of physical activity to good health has long been known, evidence continues to mount. Some evidence is highly encouraging, such as new research that shows that physical activity can help ward off and alleviate depression, and that vigorous physical activity by teenage girls can build strong bones, and prevent bone loss later in life. Some evidence is discouraging, such as one state's statistics that show that preventable chronic diseases and injuries will shorten the lives

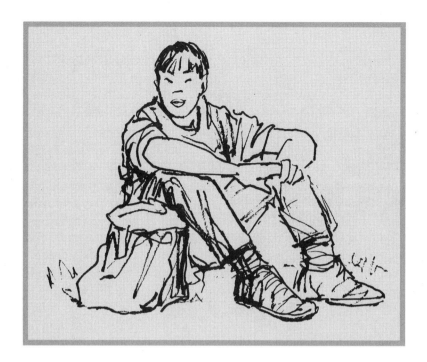

of nearly 50 percent of the children in that state. Two major factors contributing to these chronic diseases are inactivity and excess weight. Altogether, poor diet and lack of physical activity result in more deaths than alcohol, firearms, infections, poisons, irresponsible sexual behavior, motor vehicles, and illicit drug use combined.

The Bad News

- Physical inactivity is the single largest risk factor for chronic disease.
- Five percent of children in the United States are considered to have high blood pressure.
- Only six percent of children ages 13-18 have good diets (1994-96), according to a 1999 report *America's Children: Key Indicator of Well-Being.* The report indicates that the decline in nutrition is related to a decline in eating fruits and drinking milk.

A recent study conducted by the Commonwealth Fund of New York found that adolescent girls reported a lack of exercise. Even though they said they knew exercise was important, only two out of three high school girls exercised three times a week, compared to 80 percent of high school boys.

The Good News

- A regular routine of physical activity is a simple remedy for potentially serious health problems later in life.

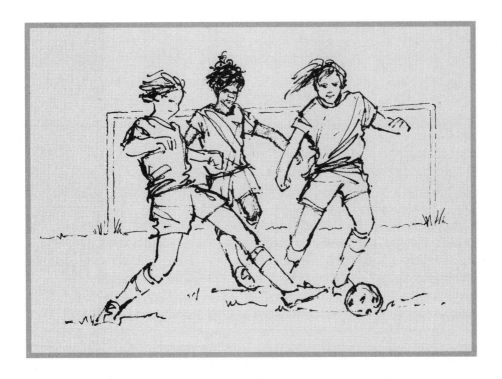

- Exercise has been shown to benefit both physical and mental health.
- Regular physical activity is great family fun. Exercising with your teens is a good thing to do, whether it is just taking a walk, sharing a game one-on-one, or spending some weekends and vacations doing outdoor activities.
- For individuals who are overweight, consistent physical activity can improve health-risk factors and self-esteem, even without weight loss.
- Weight-bearing exercises, such as walking, dancing, and jogging, can build muscle mass and help prevent osteoporosis later in life.
- It is never too late to start good health and fitness habits.

Adult Role Models

Middle and high school students need to get the serious message about the health risks of an inactive lifestyle. Teens will benefit by seeing the adults in their families enjoying physical activity as part of their everyday lives. If adults do not take positive actions for their own health and fitness, the children and teens who live with them may wonder just how important physical activity and fitness are, and draw their own conclusions that physical activity and good health are not important.

Competitive Sports

Organized sports will always be popular, and may provide a high level of fitness and well being for those who participate. Team sports also let kids see that physical fitness and skill can be important routes to self-esteem and popularity. Today more girls are participating in team sports than ever before; about 3.8 million high school boys and 2.5 million high school girls are on sports teams. Still the percentage of high school girls on sports teams remains low. In the Commonwealth Fund study, only 20 percent of high school girls said they participated in organized sports outside of gym class, compared to 59 percent of high school boys.

However, the competitive side of sports may give the message that these benefits are not for everybody. There is a danger that the overall message kids get is that physical fitness is primarily about competition, and that only the best are allowed to participate. With this focus, even student athletes run the risk of losing the motivation to seek out physical activity once their competitive careers are over.

Those who do not participate, whether it is because they are less physically gifted or just are not as interested, may turn into spectators, ready for a lifetime of watching sports on TV and from the stands.

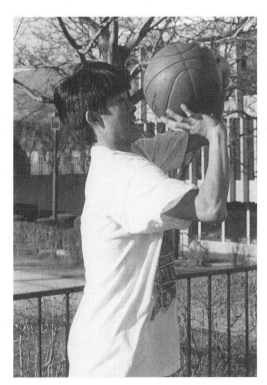

A well-used basketball hoop in the driveway and being on a basketball team can spell physical fitness, skills, popularity, and high self-esteem.

Lifetime Fitness

All teens, especially those who do not participate in organized sports, need positive messages and examples about physical activity intended to promote lifetime fitness. School physical education classes, which traditionally provided exercise and training for public school students, are now serving less than one third of high school students. Even for students who are enrolled in physical education, classes may not be long or frequent enough to provide needed levels of physical activity. Therefore, family and personal motivation is vital.

As Dr. David Rosen at the University of Michigan Medical Center advises, teens may choose to engage in individual or group activities such as walking, jogging, weight training, aerobics, hiking, bicycling, rollerblading, and swimming. They may enjoy movement disciplines such as dance, yoga, or tai chi, and martial arts such as aikido, judo, or karate. One caution for weight training: unsupervised strength training with weights or machines can result in significant harm to the musculoskeletal system in growing children. Teens should be taught correct warm-up, cool-down, stretching, and breathing techniques, as well as how to adjust equipment.

Each individual needs to find physical activities that he or she enjoys. Families and schools need to encourage every child and adolescent to do just that. The issue of lifelong health is simply too serious to allow teens to slide by without some physical activity every single day.

HEALTHY EATING

Teens are notorious for eating half meals, eating on the run, consuming large quantities of fast food, snacking on fatty, sugary, or salty foods, and for skipping meals altogether. Try not to make food a power struggle. Eating is one of the few issues over which a teen can exert control. Hopefully, the influence you have had on your teen's food habits and choices before the teen years will survive.

The core of the issue is to help your family develop healthy eating habits, not just for today, but for a lifetime. There is a link between what you eat and how you feel, how you look, and how you act, now and in later years. Eating choices are extremely important. Diet-related diseases such as heart disease, certain types of cancer, and osteoporosis (brittle bones from lack of calcium) are related to food choices.

A recent study reported in the *Journal of the American Medical Association* found heart problems in boys and girls as young as fifteen. The study looked at nearly 3,000 people who had died in accidents from 1987 to 1994. About 60 percent of the teens had fatty streaks and hard plaque signaling the onset of atherosclerosis in the coronary arteries. Autopsies done on children as early as two years old revealed fatty streaking. The American Academy of Pediatrics recommends that

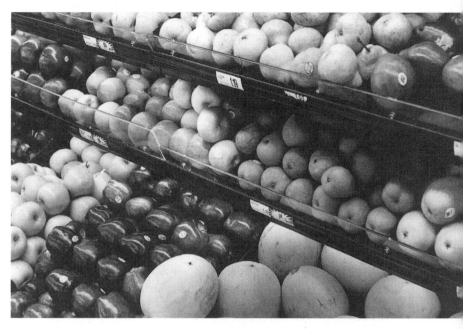

Fresh fruits and vegetables are usually abundant in grocery stores and farmers markets. They make good healthy snacks for growing teens.

initial cholesterol levels be checked as early as age two. The goal for the maintenance of a healthy heart is a cholesterol level of less than 200 mg/dl. Researchers concluded that these fatty streaks in childhood often become life-threatening plaques later on, increasing the risk of heart attack.

Teens generally do not see or care about diseases "down the road." The challenge to the person in charge of food shopping and preparation is to be creative without the family necessarily knowing that they are eating for good health!

Food for families needs to come each day from the five food groups found on the Food Guide Pyramid located at the end of this chapter. If families can possibly pay attention to the number of servings suggested for each food group, they will do fine. When you go to the grocery store, keep in mind that although prepackaged foods make life easier for busy families, they also contain more sodium (salt), refined carbohydrates, and fat than foods that you prepare yourself (besides generally costing more).

To help your family stay on a healthier diet, plan ahead so there are plenty of healthy snacks available, such as:

- Fresh fruits and vegetables—cleaned, cut, and ready to eat
- Low-fat dips
- Crackers or pretzels (choose the brands with little or no fat)
- Low-fat popcorn
- Baked chips and salsa

- Fruit juices ready to drink
- Rice cakes
- Graham crackers
- Cauliflower with reduced-calorie dressing
- Frozen fruit bars
- Nonfat blueberry yogurt
- Minestrone soup
- Mini-pack raisins
- Raisin bread with light cream cheese
- Thick-style crisp breads
- Cucumber slices with sliced mozzarella cheese

In addition to having poor eating and snacking habits, teens often skip breakfast. Research has shown that kids who do not eat breakfast do not do as well on tests in school. Their bodies have no "fuel" to go on! As an alternative, offer easy, "grab and go" foods to your teen, such as:

- A sandwich
- Cereal bars
- Fruit to go
- Pita bread or bagels
- A milk shake
- Yogurt

Food Labels

Preparing a healthy diet is getting easier. Manufacturers are required by law to label foods with their nutritional values. On each label, you will see a percentage of Daily Value listed for certain nutrients found in the food. The percent tells you how much of the maximum daily amount one serving contains. The percentages are based on the Daily Values for a 2,000-calorie diet. If a person needs fewer or more calories each day, decrease or increase the Daily Values slightly.

For Vitamins A and C, calcium, and iron, the Food and Drug Administration (FDA) considers any food that contains 10 to 19 percent of the Daily Value per serving a good source for that nutrient. If a food contains 20 percent or more of the Daily Value, it is an excellent source of the nutrient. Try to meet 100 percent of the Daily Value of these vitamins and minerals in the foods eaten each day. Bear in mind that eating too many nutrients can cause problems.

With fat (especially saturated fat), sodium, and cholesterol, you want to look for lower percentages or levels. Be aware that many foods labeled "no fat" or "low fat" may contain high levels of sugar and carbohydrates, which may result in excess calorie intake. Americans have serious health problems because of over-eating.

Here is a sample nutrition label from a package of frozen vegetables. With food labels now listing nutrition facts, you can now make a more informed choice.

Nutrition Facts

Serving Size 2/3 cup (89g)
Servings Per Container about 3

Amount Per Serving

Calories 70   Calories from Fat 5

		% Daily Value*
Total Fat 0.5g		1%
Saturated Fat 2.5g		0%
Cholesterol 0mg		0%
Sodium 105mg		4%
Total Carbohydrate 12g		4%
Dietary Fiber 4g		16%
Sugars 6g		
Protein 5g		

Vitamin A 6%	Vitamin C 15%
Calcium 0%	Iron 4%

*Percent Daily Values are based on a 2,000 calorie diet. Your daily values may be higher or lower depending on your calorie needs:

	Calories	2,000	2,500
Total Fat	Less than	65g	80g
Sat Fat	Less than	20g	25g
Cholesterol	Less than	300mg	300mg
Sodium	Less than	2,400mg	2,400mg
Total Carbohydrate		300g	375g
Dietary Fiber		25g	30g

Calories per gram:
Fat 9   Carbohydrate 4   Protein 4

Changing Needs for Growing Kids

Adolescents have increased nutrient needs because of the growth spurt that occurs during this stage of life. This growth spurt, part of puberty, usually begins for girls around ages nine to ten and for boys around the ages of eleven to twelve.

Hormonal changes and the later onset of the growth spurt in boys contribute to greater muscle and skeletal growth, requiring a higher intake of protein, iron, calcium, and zinc. In contrast, the growth spurt in girls is characterized by a smaller increase in muscle mass and a greater increase in fatty tissue. The nutritional needs for girls are therefore somewhat lower than those for boys, except girls require more iron because of the onset of menstruation.

How adolescents feel about their bodies is closely related to how they feel about themselves. The changes of puberty take place at different times for different people. The Commonwealth Fund Survey of the Health of Adolescent Girls found that more high school girls turn to dieting and counting calories rather than exercise to control weight. Only half the teen girls surveyed (53 percent) thought they were the right weight and one-third thought they were too heavy. If parent or caregivers have any indication that their son or daughter has an eating disorder related to weight control, please read the section on eating disorders located in Chapter Three for assistance.

Many teens wonder if the changes they are experiencing in their bodies are normal. Reinforce for your teens that, indeed, the changes are a natural part of growing up and that they need to take care of the body they have. Teens should be encouraged to talk about how they feel about their developing bodies with a supportive family member or a person they trust, such as a teacher, school nurse, or counselor.

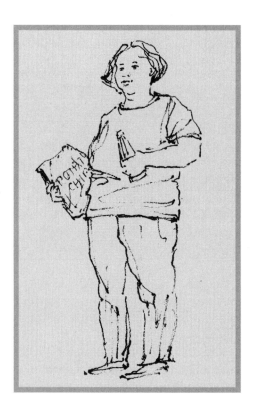

Vital Nutrients

It is important that your teen eats a relatively balanced diet from the five major food groups (see Food Guide Pyramid, located at the end of this chapter). Also, it is especially important with teens to monitor their intake of protein, calcium, iron, and total fruits and vegetables.

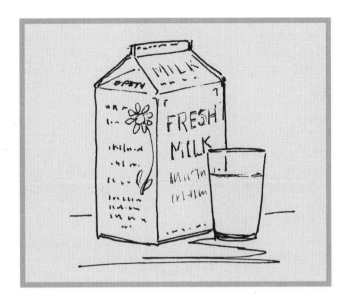

PROTEIN: Many older teenage boys (ages fifteen to eighteen) eat twice the recommended allowance of protein, or more, in the belief that a diet high in protein will give them a competitive advantage in sports. Misconceptions about the role of diet are common in the competitive world of sports. However, the basic facts are simple: Fitness and good performance require an adequate intake of calories and nutrients. With a few minor exceptions, eating enough from the five food groups on the Food Pyramid provides the proper intake; supplements and special preparations are generally unnecessary and may, in some instances, be harmful. Once the body's requirements for protein have been met, excess protein is processed just like any other excess form of calories—it is deposited as fat, not muscle. In addition, chronic excess protein consumption may have adverse effects on kidney function in the long term.

If your teen has decided to become a vegetarian, time will need to be spent making protein pairs (example: beans and rice) so he or she gets the amount of protein needed. Your library has numerous books available on healthy vegetarian eating (see REFERENCES AND RESOURCES section at the end of this chapter).

CALCIUM: As your teen's skeletal mass (size of bone structure) increases, his or her calcium requirements also increase. Girls need about 1300 mg. of calcium daily. (A cup of milk or 6 ounce container of yogurt has 300 mg. of calcium.) During the teen years, more than one-third of a person's bone mass is deposited. If calcium intake is very low, the body maintains normal blood-calcium levels by drawing calcium from the bones. This can have serious consequences: Teens may not develop optimal bone density, which may increase their susceptibility to the disease osteoporosis later in life.

Girls especially, are prone to have too low an intake of calcium throughout the teen years, largely because milk—our single best source of calcium—is so often shunned as fattening. Skim milk is a good, low-fat source of calcium—a fact surprisingly few people realize. Teens who do not drink milk should be encouraged to include other good sources of calcium listed here in their diet.

Sources of Calcium:

- Calcium-fortified foods and drinks
- Non-fat (skim) milk
- Low-fat yogurt, cheese, or cottage cheese
- Non-fat dry milk added to meat loaf or hamburgers
- Calcium-precipitated tofu
- Canned salmon and sardines that contain the bones
- Broccoli, beans and bean sprouts

Another reason for low calcium intake is the substitution of soft drinks for milk. If a fight develops over "no soft drinks in this house"—your teen will likely just get soft drinks from other sources. The trick is to think of ways to increase calcium, and it is strongly recommended that the calcium be provided in *food*, if at all possible. Check with your physician about a supplement if your teen does not drink any milk or eat any dairy products.

The high intake of soft drinks has been cited as a major contributor to childhood obesity by the U.S. Department of Agriculture and the Centers for Disease Control. Talk to your teen about how his or her health can be seriously affected by soft drinks. Suggest a voluntary limitation—one serving per day or less.

Iron: Iron helps the blood carry oxygen to the cells. People can feel tired if they become anemic from not getting enough iron in their diet. Iron requirements increase in adolescence because of the greater muscle mass and blood volume associated with the growth spurt. Refer to the Recommended Daily Allowances (RDA) chart for ages eleven to eighteen, located at the end of this chapter, to help plan for the amount your teen needs. The onset of menstruation slightly increases the iron requirements for girls. Iron found in red meats (heme iron) is absorbed more easily than iron from grains and vegetables (non-heme iron). Consumption of vitamin C along with grains and vegetables will help with the absorption of non-heme iron, and will also increase the absorption of heme iron.

Teenagers may have difficulty obtaining the recommended 12-15 milligrams of iron a day from food sources alone if their calorie intake is low. Therefore, adolescents need to consume foods with a high availability of iron, such as red meats and peanut butter, or eat combinations of good non-heme sources of iron along with foods rich in vitamin C. An example would be iron-fortified cereal with orange juice and/or an egg with orange juice. Other good sources of iron include brown rice, spinach, green peas, dried fruit, sweet potatoes and watermelon. Your physician can advise you about supplements to avoid iron deficiency anemia, if necessary.

Total fruits and vegetables: The intake of whole fruits and vegetables has been linked to cancer prevention. The cancer protection results not so much from the vitamins than it is from substances called phytochemicals that are present in fruits and vegetables.

Planning Family Meals

The Food Pyramid and the 1995 U.S. Dietary Guidelines, located at the end of the chapter, contain information that will help you in planning daily meals, and will guide your family, including your teen, toward a lifetime of healthy eating. Try to steadily adjust your family's diet toward a simple, balanced, no-nonsense routine of making healthier food choices. "The practice of good eating habits should begin as early as infancy. Children learn to develop a taste for foods they have been exposed to," says Dr. Sylmara Chatman at St. John Health System in Detroit, Michigan.

Teens also need to learn about healthy food preparation. To avoid food-borne bacteria, like listeria, teach your teen to wash all fruits and vegetables thoroughly and keep them separate from uncooked meats. Meats need to be refrigerated and cooked thoroughly. Also hands, knives and cutting boards should be washed in hot sudsy water after handling raw meats.

Feeding Your Athlete

For teen athletes, sports nutrition experts recommend eating two or three hours before a game. That means for Saturday morning games, a good breakfast is important. For late-afternoon games, breakfast, lunch and a light afternoon snack are needed. Stay away from foods that are hard to digest, such as oily, greasy foods. Eat plenty of carbohydrates and starchy foods, like breads, pasta, cereal, pancakes, or rice. Low-fat foods, such as chicken or turkey breast, are also good choices, along with low-fat milk or yogurt.

It is also important to drink plenty of liquids, one or two cups of water before exercise and another 3-6.5 ounces every ten to fifteen minutes for hot weather and high activity levels. Avoid soda, fruit drinks or juice before the game, because the sugar content can lead to stomach cramps.

Dental Health

During the teen years, many young people begin neglecting the necessary care of their teeth. When children are younger, families often take responsibility for making sure they brush and floss regularly. As they become teenagers, older family members tend to assume that kids can handle this responsibility themselves, and no longer reinforce the need for good brushing and flossing.

Teens need a reminder now and then about the importance of taking care of their teeth. Brushing teeth helps prevent plaque, a clear film that sticks to teeth and attracts bacteria that can cause cavities. Plaque can also cause the gum disease gingivitis. It is important to brush at least twice a day, after breakfast and before bed, and to spend at least three minutes brushing the fronts, sides and backs of teeth. Flossing every day and visiting the dentist twice a year are good habits teens need to practice to keep their teeth healthy.

Teens often develop extreme inflammation of the gums and an increased possibility of decay. Also, it is now known that poor gum health and the bacteria that cause gum disease can lead to problems with the heart and circulation later in life. Families often pay less attention to the diet of teens as well, so it is not unusual to see a big increase in tooth decay (cavities). Ask for advice from your dentist on how to keep track of your child's dental health, and for information on how you can help motivate your teen to take proper care of teeth and gums.

Preventing Injury to Teeth

Many teenagers are active in sports and other physical activities and, as they get older, the amount of physical contact increases. Unfortunately, injuries can and do occur in sports, and they often involve the mouth—sometimes damaging teeth for a lifetime. While teeth can usually be restored to an acceptable function and appearance, the effects of dental injury are often lifelong. In order to prevent these devastating injuries, teen athletes should wear a mouthguard during sports or physical activities.

Mouthguards have traditionally been reserved for football or hockey, but today, mouthguards are also used for basketball, soccer, and field hockey. Experts advise that both boys and girls now wear mouthguards during many sports activities. However, a recent study showed that only a small percentage of soccer players, for example, wore mouthguards. Among those who did not wear a mouthguard, one in 10 reported a dental injury; however, none of those who wore a mouthguard reported an injury. Ask your dentist to help you select a custom-fitted mouthguard that will best fit your son or daughter and adequately protect his or her teeth.

Orthodontics: A Lifetime Benefit

Orthodontics, usually called "braces," are recommended for many different reasons, and many teens need such treatment. When your dentist refers your child to the orthodontist, he or she is doing so for a specific reason. Most often, the reasons are related not so much to appearance but to the proper functioning of the teeth. Of course, after treatment they may also have nicer looking teeth due to a more correct positioning. When teeth are positioned correctly, the teeth and gums are healthier and easier to clean. These benefits will last for a lifetime.

If your son or daughter has braces, cleaning of the teeth and gums is extremely important. With wires, brackets, or appliances, it is more difficult to brush, and almost impossible to floss. Food also tends to collect on the brackets and bands, making more potential areas for decay to begin. The only solution is to take the extra time to make sure he or she maintains proper oral hygiene. This is difficult in the teenage years—a time when even toothbrushing is sometimes neglected. Both your dentist and orthodontist can help work with your teen on good home care, but they will need your participation to reinforce the importance of good dental hygiene habits.

TEENS TAKING RESPONSIBILITY FOR THEIR HEALTH

As teens become more independent, they need to learn to take responsibility for their own medical care. You can encourage this is by telling your teen about their personal health history as well as inherited diseases in the family. If your teen has a chronic illness, such as diabetes, make sure he or she knows what medications are needed and when they must be taken. Older teens who drive should be responsible for carrying their own health insurance card and for keeping doctor appointments. Adolescents need more privacy with their physician or health care provider, so remember to give them time alone for asking personal questions. Please recognize that teens usually will not discuss many health issues with their healthcare provider unless their confidentiality is assured.

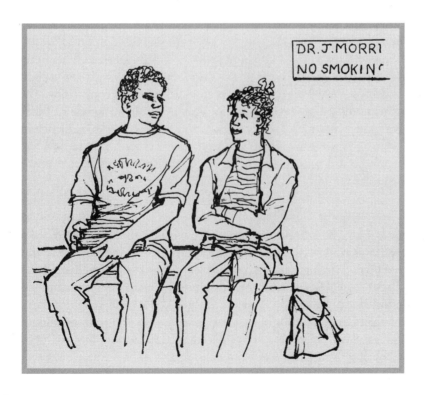

Occasionally, teens seek medical care without their parents' knowledge. Under state and federal laws, teens can seek diagnosis and treatment for sexually transmitted diseases, pregnancy, and drug abuse without parental permission.

The Commonwealth Fund Survey of the Health of Adolescent Girls found that high school girls wanted to get information from their doctor on topics such as drinking, taking drugs, sexually transmitted diseases, and eating disorders, but only one-fourth said their doctor has discussed these sensitive topics with them.

It is important that teens have trusted adults they can turn to when they need medical care and advice. In short, teens need health care providers who understand adolescent health issues. Parents and caregivers can assist their adolescents in locating health sources where teens are comfortable and know they have confidentiality. In the Commonwealth study, one-quarter of girls and one-fifth of boys said there were times they needed health care but did not receive it. One-third of these respondents said they did not want to tell their parents about the problem. Parents need to keep communication moving and show understanding, so teens will come to them with health issues.

Understanding Family Health Risks

Help your teen understand what genetic health risks your family may face. Such illnesses as diabetes, heart disease, high blood pressure, breast and colon cancer, Alzheimer's disease, depression, bipolar disorder, and multiple sclerosis often are passed on in families. Tendencies toward alcoholism or obesity can also be a part of the family picture.

You could make it a family project to research the illnesses that affected past generations in your family. Look for deaths under age 50. Then remind your teen of the need to be tested for symptoms of illness that run in your family. The point to stress is that many of these conditions can be controlled, especially if diagnosed early. You and your teens might benefit from regular checks of blood pressure, blood sugar, or cholesterol. If your teen does have a chronic health condition, such as diabetes or asthma, help him or her learn how to manage the treatment independently.

School-Based Health Clinics

The number of school health clinics has grown since the first were established in the early 1970s, and today there are more than 1,100 such clinics across the country. School-based health clinics increase access to health care by young people.

They can be very effective in offering mental health services, as well as physical health services. Such clinics provide a safe place for teens to get information on sensitive topics from a health care professional, as well as health care for common illnesses. (See REFERENCES AND RESOURCES for information on CHIP, a program for low-cost health insurance for your children.)

COMMON TEEN ILLNESSES

Strep Throat

Strep Throat is a disease caused by bacteria called Group A streptococci. It is spread when healthy people come into contact with people who have the strep bacteria in their throat. It can spread by touching, sneezing, or coughing. If teens get strep throat, they will feel sick in twelve hours to five days after being exposed to the bacteria. They will have an extremely sore, red throat with difficulty swallowing. Teens can take an over-the-counter pain reliever such as acetaminophen, to ease soreness and fever. Strep throat can also be treated with antibiotics, such as penicillin. It is important to finish all the medicine because strep throat could lead to kidney disease if inadequately treated.

Mononucleosis

Mononucleosis is caused by the Epstein-Barr virus. It is sometimes called the "kissing disease" because it is spread through direct contact with infected saliva, such as sharing a straw or eating utensil, or kissing. Teens who get this virus feel extremely tired, have a sore throat, high temperature, headache, sore muscles, and swollen lymph nodes, which are the glands located in the neck, underarms and groin. Mono also causes the liver and spleen to be swollen. There is no treatment for mono, but the disease usually goes away in one to three weeks. The best treatment is to get plenty of rest, take acetaminophen for fever and aching muscles, gargle with warm salt water, and drink plenty of water and juices. Even when your teen is feeling better, they need to take it slow. They should not participate in sports for at least a month. As long as their spleen is enlarged, there is the danger of having it rupture, requiring emergency surgery. Easy does it.

Chronic Fatigue

Most teens need at least eight hours of sleep, but many have overloaded schedules that prevent them from getting the sleep they need. They start their days early, with high school often beginning before 8 A.M. Homework, school activities, sports, and jobs often keep them up till the late hours of the night. Many teens feel tired all the time. Chronic sleep deprivation can lead to fatigue, moodiness, behavior problems, and poor academic performance. It can also put teens at risk for accidents, especially when driving or doing other tasks that demand concentration. Encourage your teen to end their day with a relaxing activity, such as a warm bath, quiet music, or reading for pleasure. Let your teen sleep in or take naps when possible. However, it is nearly impossible to "catch up" on sleep. Encourage your teen to unload his or her overloaded schedule. Excessive sleep need can be a symptom of depression or substance abuse (see related chapters).

Vaginal Infections

Teen girls need to know when they might have a vaginal infection and what to do about it. The three common vaginal infections are:

- TRICHOMONIASIS: This is caused by a parasite. There may be no symptoms at all, or there may be a smelly, greenish yellow, sometimes frothy, discharge. Most of the time trichomoniasis is contracted through intercourse. This is one of the most frequently seen sexually transmitted diseases in physicians' offices.

- YEAST INFECTIONS: Yeast is a fungus commonly found in the vagina. When the acidic balance of the vagina is upset—by such causes as antibiotics, emotional stress, tight-fitting jeans or nylon underpants— yeast can multiply and cause an infection. The symptoms include itching and a thick, white discharge. Over-the-counter medications can treat a yeast infection.

- BACTERIAL VAGINOSIS: The bacterium Gardnerella vaginalis can cause infection. The symptoms include a thick, grayish discharge, sometimes with a fishy odor. Usually there is no itching. A doctor can prescribe medicine for a bacterial vaginal infection. On occasion, the partner of your daughter may need to be treated.

It is important for your teen daughter to see a health care professional if she has a vaginal infection. Here are some ways to prevent infections:

- Wear cotton or cotton-crotch panties.
- Avoid tight-fitting clothes.
- Bathe or wash the genital area daily.
- Wipe from front to back after a bowel movement to avoid spreading bacteria to the vaginal area.
- Avoid douching. Douching is a "sure fire" way to upset the delicate balance of the vagina.

Acne

Acne is the term for plugged pores, pimples and deeper lumps that occur on the face, neck, back, chest, and shoulders. Many teens are affected by acne to some extent. The condition usually clears up after several years, but left untreated, acne can cause permanent scarring.

Acne is caused when rising hormone levels cause the oil glands of the skin to get bigger. The glands are connected to a hair-containing canal called a follicle. The oil stimulates the lining of the follicle, causing the cells of the lining to stick together and form a plug at the skin surface. The oil and cells also allow bacteria to grow, causing pimples.

Although dirt does not cause acne, it is important for your teen to wash his or her face with soap and water twice a day. Foods do not cause acne, although some people find that certain foods make their acne worse. A physician can recommend a treatment plan for acne. Treatment can include over-the-counter acne lotions, a prescription for a cream or lotion to unblock pores and reduce bacteria, or antibiotics that are applied to the skin or taken by mouth. In cases of severe acne, a dermatologist is sometimes consulted. The dermatologist has other treatment options, and sometimes might inject cortisone into the bumps to make them go away. It is important for teens to not scratch, pop or squeeze pimples, since this can lead to redness and swelling. There is no instant cure for acne but it can be controlled.

INJURY PREVENTION

Unintentional injuries are the leading cause of death for teens. Most of these injuries are preventable. Here are some ideas to prevent injuries in teens.

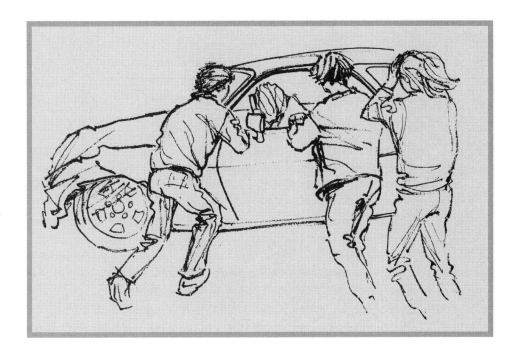

Teens and Safe Driving

Three out of 10 adolescents who die are killed in motor vehicle crashes. That amounts to more than 6,000 deaths per year, according to the National Highway Traffic Safety Administration. About one-quarter of fatal teenage crashes involve the use of alcohol or other drugs. Younger drivers, those 16-year-olds who just got their license, are three times more likely as older teens to be killed in a crash.

The following precautions can help prevent a car crash or increase chances of survival:

- Always wear a seat belt, even on short trips.
- Drive within the speed limit. Slow down when weather and road conditions are hazardous.
- If you have been drinking or using drugs, do not drive.
- Do not drive with someone who has been drinking or using drugs.
- Pay attention to your driving. Do not overload the car with passengers (distractions may cause an accident).

Teach your teen driver that vehicle maintenance is another responsibility of the driver. A car with mechanical problems can break down and result in an accident or leave your teen stranded when safety may be jeopardized. Remind your teen to regularly check the headlights, taillights, turn signals, brake lights, and tires. Drivers should know how to operate the jack and change the tire if necessary.

> Younger drivers, those 16-year-olds who just got their license, are three times more likely as older teens to be killed in a crash.

Impress upon your teen that failure to obey traffic laws can result in an accident, and a loss of their license. Posted speed limits are for ideal weather conditions. Teens need to learn to drive more slowly when it is dark, raining, or foggy, and in ice and snow. An empty parking lot is a good place to teach your teen how to handle the car on slippery pavement.

Negotiate with your teen in advance a plan to ensure their safe return from parties and other activities. It is a good idea to have your teen call you for a ride home *no questions asked* if a problem arises. You may want to discuss the issue at a later time, when your temper is under control about the incident.

Water Sports Safety

Drowning is another leading cause of death among teens. Teach your teen to always swim or boat with a partner and to never venture into water beyond their swimming ability. They need to check the depth before diving into water. Diving head-first into unexpectedly shallow water can result in a broken neck and permanent paralysis. This is a common and terrible injury among teen-age boys who may have been drinking alcohol or using other drugs. Speak to your teen about this danger. Water sports and drinking or other drugs are a dangerous combination.

Bicycling Safety

Bicycling is another common source of injury to teens. Remind your teen to observe all traffic signs, signals and pavement markings. Head injuries are a serious risk when bicycling. Your teen should wear a helmet when biking on streets, sidewalks, or bike paths. Choose helmets that meet the Snell Memorial Foundation standard for safety or the guidelines from the American National Standards Institute. Set an example by wearing a helmet yourself when you bike or use in-line skates.

In-line Skating Safety

In-line skating, or rollerblading, is one of the hottest recreational sports around. It is an excellent low-impact aerobic activity, but teens need to remember some safety tips to prevent injuries:

- Use the buddy system. Remind your teen to go with an experienced skater the first few times. Better yet, sign them up for professional instructions on striding and stopping techniques.
- Make sure they protect themselves with a helmet, pads for knees, wrists, and elbows.
- Suggest teens choose smooth, flat, wide surfaces that have few cars, bikes or pedestrians. Avoid skating at night or on wet pavement.
- Make sure your young person sees a doctor if he or she experiences popping, clicking, or swelling in the knee, hip, or ankle, even if they have not taken a fall.

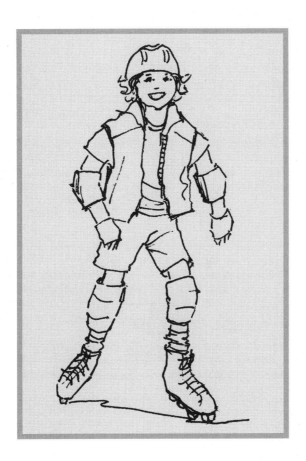

The Food Guide Pyramid

Key

● Fat (naturally occurring and added)

▽ Sugars (added)

These symbols show fat and added sugars in foods. They come mostly from the fats, oils, and sweets group. But foods in other groups—such as cheese or ice cream from the milk group, or french fries from the vegetable group—can also provide fat and added sugars.

Fats, Oils, and Sweets
Use Sparingly

Milk, Yogurt, and
Cheese Group
**2-3 Servings
5 Servings
for adolescents**

Meat, Poultry, Fish,
Dry Beans, Eggs,
and Nuts Group
2-3 Servings

Vegetable Group
3-5 Servings

Fruit Group
**2-4 Servings
2-3 Servings
for adolescents**

Bread, Cereal, Rice,
and Pasta Group
**6-11 Servings
9-11 Servings
for adolescents**

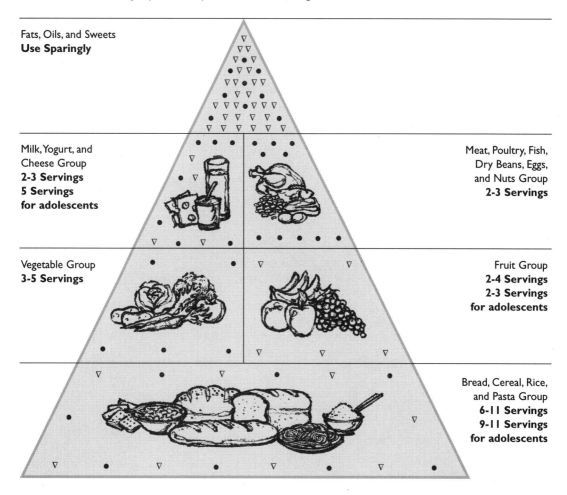

The Food Guide Pyramid emphasizes foods from the five major food groups shown in the three lower sections of the Pyramid. Noted are the special requirements for adolescents. Each of these food groups provides some, but not all, of the nutrients needed. Foods in one group cannot replace those in another. No one of these major food groups is more important than another one—for good health, all are needed.

1995 U.S. Dietary Guidelines

- Eat a variety of foods.
- Balance the food you eat with physical activity—maintain or improve your weight.
- Choose a diet low in fat, saturated fat, and cholesterol.
- Choose a diet with plenty of grain products, vegetables, and fruits.
- Choose a diet moderate in sugars.
- Choose a diet moderate in sodium (salt).

Recommended Daily Allowances Age 11 to 18

	Girls		Boys	
Nutrients	11-14 years	15-18 years	11-14 years	15-18 years
Protein (g.)	46	44	45	59
Calcium (mg.)	1300	1300	1200	1200
Iron (mg.)	15	15	12	12

REFERENCES & RESOURCES

Nutrition and Health

American Academy of Audiology: (8300 Greensboro Drive, Suite 750, McLean VA 22102. 703-790-8466, fax: 703-790-8631) Provides information about hearing, hearing aids, assistive-listening devices, and audiology services. Web site: www.audiology.org.

American Diabetes Association: (1660 Duke Street, Alexandria, VA 22314, 800-342-2383) The nation's leading nonprofit health organization, providing diabetes research, information and advocacy. Staff and volunteers in more than 800 communities conduct programs in all 50 states and the District of Columbia. The mission of the organization is to prevent and cure diabetes, and to improve the lives of all people affected by diabetes. Web site: www.diabetes.org.

The American Dietetic Association: (216 W. Jackson Blvd., Chicago, IL 60606-6995 800-877-1600) *Consumer Nutrition Hotline:* 800-366-1655. Speak to dietitians, referrals, and publications. The Chicago-based ADA is the world's largest organization of food and nutrition professionals. With nearly 70,000 members, ADA serves the public by promoting nutrition, health and well-being. Web site: www.eatright.org.

American Heart Association: (National Center, 7272 Greenville Avenue, Dallas, Texas 75231) Customer Heart and Stroke Information: 800-AHA-USA1. Brochures & information: 800-432-7854. Web site: www.americanheart.org/.

American Speech-Language-Hearing Association: (10801 Rockville Pike, Rockville MD 20852.) Answer Line: 888-321-ASHA. Action Center: 800-498-2071, 301-897-5700, 301-897-0157 (TTY), 301-571-0457 (fax). The mission of the American Speech-Language-Hearing Association is to promote the interests of and provide the highest quality services for professionals in audiology, speech-language pathology, and speech and hearing science, and to advocate for people with communication disabilities. The Web site is designed for professionals and consumers. Parents can find related brochures, self-help groups, infant hearing legislation, summer programs for children with communication disorders, and links to local certified professionals. Web site: www.asha.org.

The Commonwealth Fund Survey of the Health of Adolescent Girls (1997) and *The Health of Adolescent Boys: Commonwealth Fund Survey Findings* (1998), (The Commonwealth Fund, One East 75th Street, New York, NY 10021-2692. 212-535-0400, fax: 212-606-3500) E-mail Address: cmwf@cmwf.org. Web site: www.cmwf.org. The Commonwealth Fund undertook a survey of 6,748 adolescents, covering a broad range of health issues related to: abuse and violence, mental health, health and risky behaviors, access to health care, and communication with physicians and other health professionals. These free reports include survey highlights, charts, and fact sheets, presenting the major findings on the topics.

Food Allergy Network: (4744 Holly Avenue, Fairfax, VA 22030, 800-929-4040.) A nonprofit organization established to increase public awareness about food allergy and anaphylaxis (a life-threatening reaction), to provide education, and to advance research on behalf of all of those affected by food allergies. Send SASE for info. Web site: www.foodallergy.org.

The Food Guide Pyramid (Home and Garden Bulletin #252, U.S. Department of Agriculture, 6505 Belcrest Road, Hyattsville, MD 20782). Send stamped, self-addressed envelope.

Head Up, Eyes Forward: A Parent's Guide to Preventing Football Injuries (Michigan Department of Community Health, 800-353-8227, Web site: www.mdch.state.mi.us, 1999). This free booklet covers injury prevention for youth and high school football. The majority of football injuries could be prevented if parents and coaches were aware of the simple precautions that are outlined in this booklet. The booklet is based on a detailed report developed by the Michigan Governor's Council on Physical Fitness, which can be downloaded from the internet at the above Web site or at www.michiganfitness.org.

KidsHealth is a Web site created by medical experts of the Nemours Foundation, devoted to providing the latest health information for kids, teens, and parents. Web site: www.kidshealth.org.

See "Going in the Hospital: What a Kid Needs to Know" (kidshealth.org/kid/feel_better/
places/hospital.html) or "Eating Well While Eating Out" (kidshealth.org/teen/nutrition/menu/
eating_out.html).

Mayo Clinic Family Health Book: The Ultimate Illustrated Home Medical Reference (William Morrow and
Company, Inc, 1996, $42.50). Since its initial publication in 1990, this book has become a classic
guide to your health concerns. *The New York Times* stated, "Deserves a place on the shelf next
to the dictionary and the encyclopedia." Now revised and updated, with a new emphasis on
self-help and prevention.

The MFit Grocery Shopping Guide: Your Guide to Healthier Choices!, Nelda Mercer, Lori Mosca, and Melvyn
Rubenfire (The Cookbook Marketplace, 1997, $10.95). Total guide to which foods are the best
for you. Over 10,000 brand name foods.

National Association of the Deaf (NAD): (814 Thayer Avenue, Silver Spring MD 20910-4500. 301-587-1788,
301-587-1789 (TTY), 301-587-1791-fax, E-mail Address: NADinfo@nad.org. Web site:
www.nad.org. NAD is the oldest and largest organization representing people with disabilities
in the United States. The NAD safeguards the accessibility and civil rights of 28 million deaf
and hard of hearing Americans in a variety of areas including education, employment, health
care and social services, and telecommunications. Programs and activities include grassroots
advocacy and empowerment, captioned media, certification of American Sign Language
professionals, certification of sign language interpreters, deafness-related information and
publications, legal assistance, policy development and research, public awareness, and youth
leadership development.

National Cancer Institute: (800-422-6237) Publications, approved mammography facilities, speak to cancer
specialists. Web site: www.nci.nih.gov. Also, see http://cancernet.nci.nih.gov for Cancernet, in which
the NCI provides a wide range of accurate, credible cancer information; reviewed regularly by
oncology experts and based on the latest research.

The ParentTeen Connection (PO Box 285 Deerfield, IL 60015-0285, $18.00 for six issues, E-mail address:
ptc@parentteen.com, Web site: www.parentteen.com). Editor Barbara Cooke is a courageous
woman. She has not only gathered around her outstanding professionals to advise ParentTeen,
but she presents information in a clear-cut, frank manner. Parents, caregivers, and professionals
need this newsletter. It could be the best dollars you spend in the year 2000.

Promoting Physical Activity: A Guide for Community Action (Centers for Disease Control and Prevention,
1999, $32.00). Resource for state and local governments; transportation, health, and community
planners; exercise specialists and health professionals; community groups; businesses; schools;
colleges and universities; recreational programs and community leagues; social service
organizations; and any other professionals or volunteers who wish to promote physical
activity and healthier lifestyles in their community, agency, or organization. Web site:
www.humankinetics.com (go to products to order).

Presidential Sports Award: We Challenge You, Get Fit: A Handbook for Youth Ages 6-17, and *Physical Education:
A Performance Checklist,* Three free booklets from the President's Council on Physical Fitness
and Sports, Washington, DC, 20004.

Raising Teenagers: The Best Resources to Help Yours Succeed, John Ganz, ed. (Resource Pathways Guidebook,
1998, $24.99). The author is a school and community counselor and university professor who has
compiled the names of more than 180 books, Web sites and videotapes, then reviewed each one
on a one-to-four star rating system.

The Right Moves: A Girl's Guide to Getting Fit and Feeling Good, Tina Schwager and Michele Schuerger (Free
Spirit Press, 1998, $14.95.) This is a fun, easy-to-read guide filled with information a girl needs to
get going! From "7 Steps to Eating Right" to "Testing Your Fitness IQ," the book features quizzes,
charts, and realistic, practical advice on getting fit, inside and out. The lead author is a certified
athletic trainer; the book is very well researched and has excellent resources. Both you and your
teen will enjoy reading it.

Skating Safe!: How to Prevent In-Line Skating Injuries, Michigan Department of Community Health (Bridge Communications, Inc.) Call 800-537-5666 for copies of this pamphlet which covers all aspects of safety information for young people learning this sport.

A Teen's Guide to Going Vegetarian, Judy Krizmanic (Puffin Books, 1994, $9.99). Much more than a guide to modifying diet, this book takes pains to explain why vegetarianism is beneficial both to the individual and to the planet. Drawing on numerous resources, Krizmanic thoroughly investigates various reasons people choose not to eat meat—health benefits, ethical concerns, and environmental factors, among them. By listing organizations and newsletters of interest, she encourages readers to become actively involved in their lifestyle choice. The second part of the book tackles how to explain your switch to your parents and friends and how to manage when eating away from home. The third part is purely practical, discussing nutrition, introducing some health foods, and providing a selection of recipes.

Total Nutrition: The Only Guide You'll Ever Need from the Mt. Sinai School of Medicine, Victor Herbert and Genell J. Subak-Sharpe, ed. (St. Martin's Press, 1995, $17.95). This book replaces fads and ignorance with scientific fact, providing expert medical advice on a large variety of topics. More than 200 tables, illustrations, and sample menus give the reader clear, authoritative information. An easy-to-read, thorough, all-in-one reference book for average people—an educated approach to healthy eating.

USDA Meat and Poultry Hotline: (800-535-4555; Washington DC residents call 202-720-3333). Taped information on food safety. USDA Agricultural Research Center Web site: http://ppmq.ars. usda.gov/index.htm.

The Wellness Encyclopedia of Food and Nutrition, Sheldon Margen (Random House, 1992, $29.95). Written by a doctor, this is one of the most authoritative guides to shopping and eating for better health and longer life.

The Yale Guide to Children's Nutrition, William V. Tamborlane, ed. (Yale University Press, 1997, $18.00). Over 100 physicians, dietitians, nurses and social workers at the Yale-New Haven Children's Hospital— as well as famous chefs from around the country—offer information about nutrition for children at each stage of development from infancy through adolescence. They provide reassuring and practicable advice that takes into account variations among families and individual children. Advice for feeding a vegetarian child, a sick child, a child athlete, and an adolescent with acne. The authors help with eating disorders, childhood obesity, cystic fibrosis, diabetes, food allergies, and attention deficit hyperactivity disorder.

Preparation of Food

Healthy Food, Healthy Soul: African American Cooking, Gabrielle Tibbs. (Michigan Department of Community Health). To order, call 800-353-8227 (one copy free). Highly recommended.

Heart Smart Cookbook, by Henry Ford Heart and Vascular Institute/Henry Ford Health System and The Detroit Free Press (*Detroit Free Press,* 1991, $14.95). Heart Smart is a community-oriented health promotion program, which tries to help the consumer become aware of how choices in food and lifestyle can affect health. This cookbook gives basic guidelines, practical tips and easy recipes that can help you live a more Heart Smart way without much fuss.

High Fit-Low Fat Cookbook and *High Fit-Low Fat Vegetarian Cookbook,* Lizzie Burt et. al. (The University of Michigan Medical Center, P.O. Box 363, Ann Arbor, Michigan 48106-0363, 800-433-MFIT, $14.95). If you think healthy recipes are boring, these books will change your mind.

The Meatless Gourmet: Favorite Recipes from Around the World, Bobbie Hinman (Prima Publishing, 1994, $15.95). Vegetarian cuisine can easily get boring, but not so with Hinman's international recipes. In this exciting book, she offers more than 350 recipes from renowned food regions like India, Mexico, Italy, the Middle East, Asia, the Caribbean, and Eastern Europe. Includes side dishes, breads and desserts to go with the main dishes. With nutritional analysis.

Moosewood Restaurant Low-Fat Favorites, The Moosewood Collective (Clarkson Potter, 1996, $22.00).
More than 250 lean recipes (many dishes get the fat down to a modest 16-17% of their total
calories) for homey, hearty food with bold, pan-ethnic flavors that have won the Moosewood
Collective cookbooks so many fans. Except for chapter on fish, most recipes are vegetarian.

Moosewood Restaurant Daily Special: Soup and Salad Combos for Every Day, The Moosewood Collective
(Clarkson Potter, 1999, $24.00). Just coming out in print.

The New Laurel's Kitchen: A Handbook for Vegetarian Cookery and Nutrition, Carol Flinders, Brian Ruppenthal,
and Laurel Robertson (Ten-Speed Press, 1996, $19.95).

The Simply Healthy Lowfat Cookbook, University of California at Berkeley (Health Letter Associates, 1995,
$24.95). (Health Letter Associates, Department 1108, 632 Broadway, New York NY 10012.)
By the editors of the Wellness Cooking School and the UCB Wellness Letter, published
by Rebus Inc. Over 250 lowfat recipes rich in the antioxidant vitamins that keep you healthy.

Simply Vegan: Quick Vegetarian Meals, Debra Wasserman, Reed Mangels (The Vegetarian Resource Group,
1999, $12.95). With over 50,000 copies sold, this is not a book that lies on the shelf but is
regularly used by busy people trying to live a vegan or vegetarian lifestyle. Over 160 good-
tasting, but quick, practical recipes are profiled. In addition, Reed Mangels gives readers a
complete vegan nutrition section that includes easy-to-read charts, menus, and meal plans.

Vegetarian Express: Easy, Tasty and Healthy Menus in 28 Minutes (or Less!), Nava Atlas and Lillian Kayte.
(Little Brown & Co., 1995, $15.95). More than one hundred and eighty recipes for low-fat,
nutritious, meatless meals. The book is divided into sections on grains, pastas, sandwiches,
and more, including recipes for side dishes to compliment each entree.

Puberty

Health 'n Me©: A Comprehensive Health Curriculum, Alice R. McCarthy (Sopris West, 4093 Specialty Place,
Longmont, Colorado 80504, 1997). This comprehensive K-6 health curriculum was written by
the author of *Healthy Teens* in close collaboration with a group of health professionals from
across the nation. Several *Michigan Model for Comprehensive School Health* lessons were used with
permission as a base for some of the lessons in *Health 'n Me.* This curriculum addresses pressing
health topics, utilizes many instructional approaches, and is built upon a solid research base.
Please see Appendix 2 for *Michigan Model* modules offered at middle and high school.

Keys to Your Child's Healthy Sexuality, Chrystal de Freitas (Barron's Educational Series, 1998, $6.95). An
experienced pediatrician and educator, who is also a parent, offers advice on how to talk
about the facts of life and sexuality to children of all ages from preschoolers through preteens.
The author recognizes that bringing up children today is different—and in many ways more
difficult—than it was in past generations.

Period (Revised with a removable Parent's Guide) Joann Gardner-Loulan, Bonnie Lopez and Marcia
Quackenbush (Volcano Press, 1991, $9.95) National Science Teacher's Association says,
"this is perhaps the only satisfactory book on this important topic."

The Period Book: Everything You Don't Want to Ask (But Need to Know), Karen and Jennifer Gravelle
(Walker and Company, 1996, $8.95). Written with her fifteen-year-old niece, the Gravelles
talk to the young girls themselves.

The Society for Adolescent Medicine (1916 Cooper Oaks Circle, Blue Springs MO 64015, 816-224-8010,
E-mail address: socadmed@gvi.net). Information on locating a specialist in your area in the field
of adolescent medicine can be obtained from this source.

Teenage Health Care : The First Comprehensive Family Guide for the Preteen to Young Adult Years, Gail B. Slap
and Martha M. Jablow (Pocket Books, 1994, $14.00). This comprehensive manual offers general
chapters on puberty, exercise, and nutrition, followed by information on a wide variety of specific
health matters from headaches to cancers. One of the best portions of the book alerts parents
to important psychological and behavioral issues that teens may face—drug abuse, depression,
learning disorders, sexual abuse, and pregnancy—providing medical background as well as an idea

of the choices and challenges such problems bring. Includes a helpful resource listing and provides a strong sense of how the health concerns confronting today's young adults differ from those of the last generation.

Your Child's Emotional Health: Adolescence, Jack Maguire/Philadelphia Child Guidance Center Staff (Macmillan Publishing Company, Inc., 1995, $9.95). One of the country's leading child psychiatric centers offers authoritative guidance to adolescent behavior and emotional development, addressing such topics as popularity, depression, discipline, sexuality, substance abuse, running away, and overeating. This book explains how to distinguish normal from troubled behavior, advising parents how to handle both ordinary and severe problems at home and when to seek professional help. This is truly an exceptional book that caring families will want to access. They will also want to know about the clinic as a resource if their child needs diagnosis and therapy.

What's Going on Down There?: Answers to Questions Boys Find Hard to Ask, Karen Gravelle (Walker & Co., 1998, $8.95). Great introductory book for ages 9-12, with a friendly style of explaining the ins and outs of puberty. Small and easy to read, with humorous illustrations.

SEE ALSO THE RESOURCES ON ADOLESCENT DEVELOPMENT FOUND IN CHAPTERS 1 AND 4.

CHAPTER 6
TEENS: SUBSTANCE ABUSE

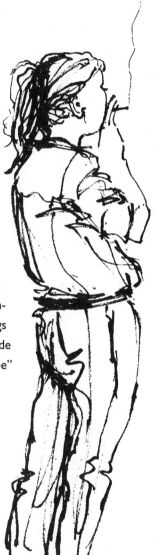

This chapter provides a wealth of current information and statistics regarding substance abuse among youth. Hopefully, this information will serve as a wake-up call to adults that substance abuse is a very real and dangerous presence in the daily lives of adolescents, both in their home settings and in the larger community. The substances discussed in this chapter include tobacco, alcohol, marijuana, heroin, cocaine, inhalants, ecstasy, and "date rape" substances.

FACTS ABOUT DRUG USE

Adults need to know the facts about drug use among teens. The statistics that directly follow are from the 24th annual *Monitoring the Future* study, a series of annual surveys of some 50,000 students in over 422 public and private secondary schools nationwide:

- 29 percent of eighth graders used an illegal drug in 1998.
- 45 percent of 10th graders used an illegal drug in 1998.
- 54 percent of 12th graders used an illegal drug in 1998.

Lloyd D. Johnston, Ph.D., the principal investigator of the study, believes illicit drug use among this age group is finally starting to decline after six years of steady increases. "The improvement so far is very modest," he said. "But at least the troublesome trends observed through most of the nineties have begun to reverse direction." Some experts believe school health education programs, and more involvement by parents and community leaders, may have prompted this turnaround. Other groups, like the federal Substance Abuse and Mental Health Services Administration, warn parents not to let their guard down. According to SAMHSA, an estimated 77,000 teenagers under the age of 18 were admitted to substance abuse centers in 1996—compared to about 44,000 teenagers in 1991.

TOBACCO

Is tobacco use among teenagers finally on a downward trend? Johnston noted in his study that all three grade levels reported a small decline in tobacco use between 1997 and 1998. "Early indications of a turnaround were evident last year," he said. "In 1997, eighth- and 10th-grade students began to show very slight improvements, even though use among 12th-graders was still rising. This year all three grade levels, encompassing young people aged 13 to 18, show some drop in smoking."

In 1998, current smoking rates were 19 percent among eighth graders (13-14 years old), 28 percent among 10th-graders (15-16 years old), and 35 percent among 12th-graders (17-18 years old).

> According to Lloyd Johnston, Smoking cigarettes usually comes before smoking marijuana, teaching teens how to take smoke into their lungs for a drug-induced effect.

These rates are impressively high, especially when compared to the fact that about 25 percent of all adults are classified as current smokers, according to the National Health Interview Survey.

Aside from the well-known risks of tobacco use, experts like Johnston believe that cigarette smoking is strongly tied to smoking marijuana. Smoking cigarettes usually comes before smoking marijuana, teaching teens how to take smoke into their lungs for a drug-induced effect. Teens who smoke cigarettes already know how to get high when it comes to smoking marijuana. Johnston and others believe that the rise in cigarette smoking may well have contributed to the rise in marijuana use.

Smoking: From Middle School on to College

One concern in particular is that only half the eighth-graders (54 percent) in Johnston's study see a "great risk" in smoking a pack-a-day of cigarettes. "That's virtually a question with a right-or-wrong answer, and nearly half of these 13- and 14-year olds get it wrong," he said. "By 12th grade, 71 percent of the students see 'great risk' in pack-a-day smoking, but by then the horse may already be out of the barn—many are already smoking."

Once your teen starts smoking, it is indeed hard to stop. A new study by the Harvard School of Public Health finds smoking rose from 22 percent to 28 percent on college campuses between 1993 and 1997. The authors believe most of this increase came from the rise in high school smoking during the early 1990s. The study found increased smoking rates in all groups, regardless of sex or race, at all colleges.

Another study, by the Centers for Disease Control and Prevention, shows overall smoking rates increased by one-third among high school students between 1991 and 1998. The same study shows an especially sharp increase in tobacco use among black teenagers over the past several years. One explanation is exposure to cigarette ads. Another reason—African American teenagers themselves say that the nicotine tends to enhance their marijuana high. Nearly 23 percent of African American teenagers surveyed in the study listed themselves as cigarette smokers, compared to 13 percent in 1991. Overall, however, Asian, African American and Hispanic students report much lower smoking rates than white students do.

Genetic Damage from Smoking

There are plenty of reasons for your teen not to smoke. A study at the University of California indicates that smoking during childhood or adolescence might cause permanent genetic damage, leading to increased risk of lung cancer, even after the smoker quits. The study analyzed 143 lung cancer patients and looked for alterations in the deoxyribonucleic acid (DNA) that are caused by tobacco and linked to cancer. It discovered that even in ex-smokers, the highest level of DNA alterations were found in those who started smoking at a young age, regardless of when they quit. According to the study, about one-third of all smokers ultimately die from a smoking-related disease such as cancer or emphysema.

Cigar Smoking

It seems harmless because it is not inhaled, but cigar smoking carries its own set of risks. Cigar sales zoomed up 44 percent between 1993 and 1998. A recent study from the American Heart Association indicates that regular cigar smoking nearly doubles the risk of cancer and circulatory problems. Researchers say the biggest danger is the risk of cardiomyopathy—deterioration of the heart muscle that erodes its ability to pump blood. Large doses of nicotine and other toxic compounds can severely damage organs of the body. Cigar smoking can do all this damage without being inhaled.

Unlike the growing campaign against cigarette smoking, the media tend to portray cigar smoking in a positive light, linking it with celebrities, money, power, fine food and wine. According to San Francisco's Institute for Health Policy Studies, a survey of 400 cigar-related stories last year found that 63 percent of the articles were generally positive about cigar smoking, while only 13 percent brought attention to the health risks.

Discussing the Facts about Tobacco Use

There are two vital issues adults need to face about teen tobacco use. First, if you do not use tobacco, you cannot assume your teen will follow suit. Second, if you do use tobacco, your teen is statistically more likely to also use tobacco. If you are a tobacco user, be straightforward with your teen about your own use. Point out the reasons you started using tobacco and be prepared to admit that you are addicted to nicotine. If you have smoked in the past but quit, talk with your teen about the addictive nature of tobacco and how hard it was to quit.

If you do not use tobacco, talk about how difficult it was to resist starting when you were a teen. Many people find it easiest to talk about the short-term effects of tobacco use first—the high cost, smelly clothes, bad breath, and yellowing teeth.

> If you have smoked in the past but quit, talk with your teen about the addictive nature of tobacco and how hard it was to quit.

You may wish to discuss the following facts as well:

- Tobacco use is considered a gateway drug to other drug use.
- Tobacco use immediately affects the user's lung capacity, especially in terms of being able to participate in athletics.
- Tobacco users have more coughs and illnesses than non-users.
- Most people do not use tobacco.
- Tobacco is becoming much less acceptable at school, in the workplace, and in public places.

Cigarette use is the most avoidable cause of death in the United States. Whether you smoke or not, you can raise a teen who does not. You need to work out rules about tobacco use with your teen to keep your teen tobacco free.

ALCOHOL

The level of drinking among teenagers has hardly changed over the last decade. For example, 14 percent of eighth-graders in the 1998 *Monitoring the Future* survey reported having five or more drinks in the last two weeks, compared to 13 percent in 1991. The use of alcohol among teens had been going up over the past few years, due in part to the increased popularity of binge drinking. But 1998 marked a slight decline in alcohol use at all three grade levels.

- 25 percent of eighth-graders reported they had "been drunk" at least once in the last year, down from 26 percent in 1997.
- 47 percent of 10th-graders reported they had "been drunk" at least once in the last year, down from 49 percent in 1997.

- 63 percent of 12th-graders reported they had "been drunk" at least once in the last year, down from 64 percent in 1997.

One explanation for this downturn could be that more teens are learning about the risks of binge drinking. Even so, Johnston notes that fully 33 percent of 12th-graders report being drunk at least once in the 30-day period before the survey. Obviously, adults who care about adolescents have their work cut out for them.

Driving While Under the Influence

Drinking and driving is the leading cause of death for teenagers 15 and older. An amazing 40 percent of all deaths in that age group are from car crashes. That's more than all diseases, homicide and suicide. Unfortunately, it seems that fewer and fewer teenagers are getting the message. For example, a recent study showed that 18 percent of high school seniors reported drinking and driving in 1997, up from 15 percent in 1995.

The same study, which surveyed about 17,000 high school seniors at 135 schools, also found that the percentage of students reporting any alcohol use in the prior month decreased from 70 percent in 1984 to slightly over 50 percent in 1995, and then rose again to 57 percent in 1997.

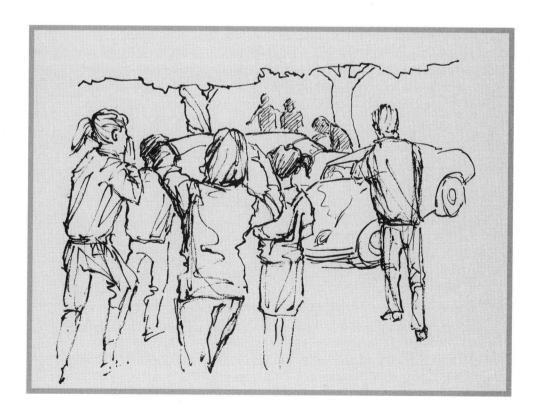

Alcohol consumption comprises a massive complex of issues that, on one hand, seems to point toward socializing, fun and good times; on the other hand, it points toward violent deaths, shattered lives and the loss of potential. Recovering alcoholics talk about their lives "performed" on the stage, under the lights of a play called "Death on the Installment Plan."

Like their elders, American teens drink at a high rate. Children as young as eight and nine list alcohol as a problem in their lives, whether the problem is caused by the drinking done by other people in their lives, or by their own drinking.

You can drink moderately yourself and raise a teen that does not drink. Your role as a parent and adult supports such a stance. The law, and the often fatal mistakes teens make while drunk or drinking, support such a stance. There is nothing hypocritical about telling your teen that alcohol is something that he or she might enjoy as an adult—but is simply not allowed now. Ask yourself, "What would you tell a 14-year-old who wants to drive your family car?"

If you drink, explain to your teen why you drink, and take some time to look at your own drinking habits. As with most behavior, teens are often better observers than they are listeners. Your drinking habits will definitely influence your teen. The old adage, "What you do speaks so loudly, I cannot hear what you say," still holds true.

Binge Drinking

Dying to take a drink? The problem of binge drinking has become so serious on the college campus that in 1998 the American Medical Association and Robert Wood Johnson Foundation, a health-care philanthropy, teamed up to study binge drinking at six different universities. Binge drinking is when a person drinks five or more alcoholic beverages in a row. One result of drinking large amounts in a short time is alcohol poisoning, in which the part of the brain that causes breathing is paralyzed, causing the victim to die of hypoxia or lack of oxygen to the brain.

In a recent survey of 14,500 college students at 116 institutions, four out of five fraternity members said they are regular binge drinkers.

Binge drinking at colleges and universities is a serious problem that needs to be confronted by each adult concerned with the lives of teens. Studies indicate that half the college binge drinkers began to drink in high school. One example of this problem is when high school seniors attend a fraternity or sorority party, where they see binge drinking and perceive it "as normal." In a recent survey of 14,500 college students at 116 institutions, four out of five fraternity members said they are regular binge drinkers. Well-publicized accounts of college students who drank too much and died from alcohol poisoning have prompted several fraternities and sororities to consider alcohol-free environments for their members.

Students about to go off to college should be cautioned about checking out the drinking practices in various sororities and fraternities before they consider joining one. Another option for parents and institutions to consider is to place freshman college students in dormitories rather than allowing them to live in fraternity or sorority houses for their first year away from home. Certainly it is important to talk with authorities at the institution of your student's choice about their policies regarding binge drinking.

Dr. Henry Wechsler, director of College Alcohol Studies at the Harvard School of Public Health says, "Most parents aren't teaching their kids anything about alcohol, especially not that alcohol in large quantities has many dangerous effects. Too many kids think that as long as they don't drive, it is O.K. to get drunk." Dr. Wechsler said parents also could help monitor the activities of their state and municipal alcohol control boards with regard to enforcement of the minimum drinking age, sales of alcohol around college campuses and bars that offer students "specials"—high volumes of alcohol (usually beer) for a low price—which he said encourage binge drinking.

Male athletes in college tend to binge drink more than any other student group. A 1998 study by the Journal of American Health revealed that 60 percent of all male athletes said they had participated in binge drinking within two weeks of the survey. High school athletes are particularly vulnerable, since they assume they are under pressure to win, perform well, and "look cool." Coaches need to get involved. Do not ignore the smell of marijuana or alcohol on an athlete. Emphasize the negative performance on the field that is caused by using drugs or alcohol. Sign a pledge with your athletes for a drug-free and alcohol-free environment. This will demonstrate support and show you are making a commitment too.

Parents tend to believe that their teens drink because of peer pressure. But more than 50 percent of students said "getting drunk" and simply having a good time is the major motivating factor in drinking, along with stress and boredom. What can parents do to keep their teens from binge drinking? One solution is to make a drug-free and alcohol-free pact with your teens through high school and college. Constantly remind them about the dangers of drugs and alcohol, and suggest other ways of dealing with stress and emotional problems. (For information see chapter three on emotional issues and stress reduction.)

Sending an Alcohol Message via the Media

Alcohol and television sometimes seem to go hand in hand. A 1999 study at Cornell University reports that actors and actresses are seen drinking alcohol on more than 40 percent of the network shows. Overall, the study found that alcohol was consumed 555 times in 224 hours of prime time television. About seven percent of the scenes involving alcohol included teenagers between the ages of 13 and 18. Another study, by the American Medical Association, shows that by the time a teenager has reached the ninth grade, he or she has probably seen more ads for beer and wine coolers than for any other product. Considering the average teenager spends more time watching television than attending school, and that the average household has television turned on for more than seven hours a day, parents need to consider the types of messages their teen is receiving.

Marijuana

The 1998 *Monitoring the Future* study found that marijuana use is leading the way in the rise of drugs among teens. In 1998, nearly 25 percent of all eighth-graders said they tried marijuana, while about 50 percent of all 12th-graders said they smoked marijuana at least once in the past year. Nevertheless, there was a slight decline in marijuana use at all three grade levels.

- 22.2 percent of all eighth-graders smoked marijuana last year, down from 22.6 percent in 1997.
- 39.6 percent of all 10th-graders smoked marijuana last year, down from 42.3 percent in 1997.
- 49.1 percent of all 12th-graders smoked marijuana last year, down from 49.6 percent in 1997.

Even more encouraging, the number of high school seniors who report smoking marijuana in the last month dropped from 23.7 percent to 22.8 percent, while the number of eighth-graders dropped from 10.2 percent to 9.7 percent. Tenth-graders report an even greater decline: 18.7 percent said they smoked marijuana in the last month, compared with 20.7 percent in 1997.

> As a parent and as an adult you need to focus on the facts about marijuana today, your family values, and what the world is like for teens today.

Johnston said he believes perceived risk factors and disapproval from friends play an important role in whether your teen will begin smoking marijuana. One especially encouraging sign is the decline of marijuana smoking among eighth-graders for the second year in a row, meaning younger students may finally be beginning to understand its harmful effects. Most teenagers say they started smoking marijuana at age 14.

Marijuana Today

For many adults, their own past marijuana use is a barrier to talking with their teen about marijuana today. The choices you made when you were young are just that—choices made in the past. As a parent and as an adult you need to address this issue in the present tense, and focus on the facts about marijuana today, your family values, and what the world is like for teens today.

Consider the following basic facts about marijuana:

- Marijuana today has much higher levels of THC (the chemical that produces the high) than before, especially compared to marijuana available in the 1960s.
- Faulty judgment while using marijuana puts teens at increased risks for automobile accidents, unplanned and unsafe sexual practices, drowning, falls, and even suicide.
- Marijuana use may slow sexual development.
- Teens who smoke pot are at an increased risk for cancer. One study found that one marijuana cigarette produced the same lung damage as five tobacco cigarettes.
- Teens who smoke marijuana are more likely to smoke cigarettes, use other drugs, and drink alcohol.

Most teens—and most adults—are familiar with marijuana. The general softening stance of many adults, teens, and society as a whole has been well documented. The huge rise in marijuana use among teens is well recorded. Few people, however, seem willing to confront the facts: Your teen may already be getting high. Your teen is being or will be offered a chance to get high and to use other drugs. Parents need to somehow marry those facts with what they really want for their son and daughter. Parents and caregivers need to take a stand today, recognizing the basic facts about teens and drugs.

HEROIN

This highly addictive drug has become more popular with high school students in recent years. Johnston's *Monitoring the Future* study indicates that 2.1 percent of high school students used heroin at least once in 1998, compared to 1.8 percent in 1996. One reason for heroin's popularity is that it is cheaper to buy and easier to find in recent years, especially in suburban neighborhoods. A second reason is that heroin and other similar street drugs are generally purer today, which allows teenagers to snort the drug rather than "shooting up" or injecting it into their blood stream. Teens believe sniffing heroin is less dangerous. But in fact the opposite is true. Users tend to misjudge the amount of heroin when sniffing it, which is one reason why the number of overdoses has jumped 53 percent since 1993. Even more disturbing is the fact that heroin use among adolescents is more prevalent today than ever. A study by the National Institute on Drug Abuse (NIDA) indicates that 8th-graders reported a higher use of heroin last year than did all older students. According to the study, the average age of a heroin user was 27 in 1998; by 1996, it had dropped to 19.

One of the most detrimental long-term effects of heroin is addiction itself. Addiction is a chronic, relapsing disease, characterized by compulsive drug seeking and use, and by neurochemical and molecular changes in the brain. Heroin also produces profound degrees of tolerance and physical dependence, which are also powerful motivating factors for compulsive use. As with abusers of any addictive drug, heroin users gradually spend more and more time and energy obtaining and using the drug. Once they are addicted, the heroin users' primary purpose in life becomes seeking and using drugs. The drugs literally change their brains. Medical consequences of chronic heroin abuse include scarred and/or collapsed veins, bacterial infections of the blood vessels and heart valves, abscesses (boils) and other soft-tissue infections, and liver or kidney disease. Of course, sharing of infected equipment or fluids can lead to some of the most severe consequences of heroin use—infections with hepatitis B and C, HIV, and a host of other blood-borne viruses.

COCAINE

Cocaine, also known as coke, toot, blow, rock, or snow, is made from coca leaves. It can be powerfully addictive. People snort it, smoke it, or inject it.

"Freebase" is a form of cocaine that is smokable. Freebasing is extremely dangerous because the drug reaches the brain in seconds and gives an intense high. When small lumps or shavings of freebase cocaine are smoked, it is known as crack.

Cocaine stimulates the central nervous system, which is why users usually have dilated pupils and are hyper when they are high. Users' hearts beat very fast when they do cocaine. The drug causes blood vessels to narrow at the same time they are trying harder to handle the additional flow of blood pumped by the heart. Body temperature and blood pressure rise, which could cause a heart attack, stroke, or seizures. Very high doses of cocaine also can cause the lungs to stop working.

Sometimes cocaine users report feeling depressed when they are not high. Other side effects include irritability, anxiety, and paranoia. Studies have shown that cocaine also may make someone, even an occasional user, violent or suicidal.

Crack and freebase cocaine are more dangerous than regular cocaine because they act faster and are more potent. Lung damage, brain seizures, and heart attacks are more likely with freebase rock.

Teenagers are still continuing to use both crack cocaine and powder cocaine. In Johnston's study, there was a slight increase of crack cocaine use among the lower grades in 1998, while the use of powder cocaine has leveled off. Perceived risks for crack cocaine, still declining in the upper grades, has at least begun to level off at eighth grade. Johnston said that's an "encouraging sign" for the future.

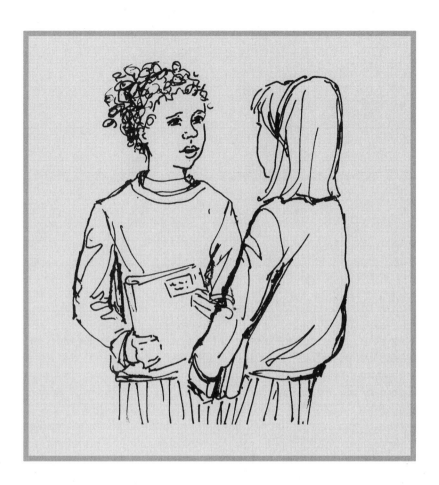

INHALANTS

There are no adult dealers pushing these substances. Kids learn about them from friends. They are legal, cheap, and easy to find. These drugs are inhalants—hundreds of household products, from cooking sprays to upholstery protectors, contain gases kids can sniff (or "huff") for a cheap high.

They are so common that you might not be alarmed if you saw a child buying them, but they can harm internal organs, cause severe brain damage, and kill the first or the 100th time they are used with what is called Sudden Sniffing Death.

Most huffers are in eighth through 12th grade, and use among kids has more than doubled since 1991. One study found that 20 percent of kids have tried it by eighth grade, yet 85 percent of parents said their children would never do such a thing.

> ## The Warning Signals for Inhalant Use:
> - Chemical smell on clothing
> - Tremors
> - Hearing loss
> - Memory loss
> - Red eyes
> - Runny nose
> - Sores around the mouth

Johnston believes a strong campaign against inhalants launched by the Partnership for a Drug-Free America has led to its declined use since 1996. Awareness by parents and education in schools must continue.

ECSTASY

This drug gained increased popularity in the 1990s. Ecstasy, or MDMA (methylenedioxymethamphetamine) stimulates the central nervous system and causes hallucinogenic effects. It has been shown to cause brain damage in animals because it can deplete an important chemical in the brain called serotonin, which affects everything from mood swings to sleeping habits. It is a synthetic drug that is swallowed, snorted, smoked or injected. Teens have been known to take Ecstasy and other "designer drugs" at all-night dance parties called raves. This combination of drugs and non-stop dancing can easily cause exhaustion and dehydration, leading to serious heart problems.

'DATE RAPE' DRUGS

There are two drugs that have recently received much media and government attention for being used to facilitate sexual assaults. Rohypnol (roofies, forget-me drug, forget pill) and Gamma Hydroxybutyrate or GHB (easy lay, Georgia Home Boy) are both powerful central nervous system depressants. Side effects include drowsiness, headaches, memory impairment or amnesia, and possible coma-like deep sleep. In 1996, Congress passed the Drug-Induced Rape Prevention and Punishment Act, providing for harsh penalties for using such drugs to commit crimes against another person. In 1999, the Drug Enforcement Administration has documented more than 4,000 cases involving overdoses of GHB, and 32 deaths.

The most common method for criminal intent is to spike someone's drink with the substance, since it is difficult to detect in this way. The best suggestion, for the person who may legally consume alcohol, is to never leave your drink unattended, and do not accept a drink from a stranger unless you watch it being poured. Individuals should never drink anything with an unusual taste or appearance, such as a salty taste or unexplained residue. If a person thinks they have been given either of these drugs, they should seek medical assistance at once and report the situation to the police.

References and Resources section is found at the end of Chapter 7.

Chapter 7
The Answer to Substance Abuse

Even when adults have accurate and up-to-date information about substance abuse among adolescents, they may believe there is little they can do to make an impact on youth, whether in their role as parents or as members of the community at large. This chapter discusses some recent studies that show that adults' actions can and do make a difference. Specific strategies are presented for the family, for teen party settings, and in support of health education in schools.

Parents and Caregivers: Crucial Players

The best way for parents and caregivers to combat substance use is to keep their teens from using drugs in the first place. A 1998 study by the Partnership for a Drug Free America indicates that talking to your teen about the dangers of drug use is the most effective strategy to achieve this goal. The study surveyed over 9,000 teenagers and 810 parents. It found that teens who receive a strong anti-drug message at home are 42 percent less likely to use drugs than other teenagers whose parents ignore the issue. At the same time, only 27 percent of the teens said they learned about drug use at home. About 98 percent of the parents said they talked about drug use with their children at least once, but only 48 percent recall having a conversation with their teen about drugs in the past year.

Parents need to understand what is happening in their teen's world. For example, only 37 percent of the parents surveyed said they thought their teen had ever been offered marijuana—but 53 percent of the teens said they were offered it. About 45 percent of the teens using marijuana said they learned nothing about drug use at home. In comparison, among the number of teens who learned a lot about drug use at home, smoking marijuana drops to 26 percent.

How Adults Can Help

Teenagers themselves say parents and caregivers can help curb drug use by sending a strong message at home. Here are some suggestions from teenagers that were raised at a recent community coalition meeting on drug use:

- Set consequences for your teen's actions. Do not allow him or her to think they are "getting away" with behavior that's unacceptable to the family.
- Discuss expectations with your children; then work with them to meet those expectations.
- If you overreact to bad news of drug use by teens in your community, you are likely not to get a full story when you bring up the issue the next time. Keep communication open and flowing about drug use in your community.

Lloyd D. Johnston, Ph.D., principal investigator of the *Monitoring the Future* study, that reports on drug use among teens, is a strong advocate of the power of families, communities, and society as a whole to reduce drug use among teens. "Each new generation needs to learn the same lessons about drugs if they are going to be protected from them," says Johnston. In short, the answer to "generational forgetting" is education and prevention. Parents, caregivers, school programs that include health education, and community leaders are the key players in reinforcing the lessons.

A FAMILY MODEL

Many families today are working with their teen to prevent drug use, whether the drug is nicotine, marijuana, alcohol, inhalants, or any other kind of drug. The model these families are using is inclusive: No drug of any kind is acceptable. This model involves the teen in the reasoning and decision-making process, and focuses on clear-cut rules and consequences. The line these adults have decided to walk goes beyond simply forbidding drug use with words and threats. The adults know the realities of drug use among teens, the temptations teens face, and show a willingness to have a relationship with their teen that makes "no drug use" work for both the families and their teen.

- Drugs are dangerous. What is known about drug use among teens points to disaster, whether the result is a life-long addiction to cigarettes or an early death in an alcohol-related traffic accident. There is absolutely no evidence to show that drug use in teens is not dangerous; rather, it is getting more dangerous. A fight when high or drunk could lead to a shooting; having sex in the same condition could lead to pregnancy or a sexually transmitted disease.

- Drug use is illegal. Adults need to know the laws in their state and lean on these laws when setting rules about drug use with their teen. Quoting laws might seem hypocritical to some people, or at least not a very sound argument, but the facts are the facts. At the very least, teens need to know that parents or other adults may be held responsible for their teen's drug or alcohol use, and for the teen's actions while under the influence of drugs. Parents, not just teens, are the ones who bear the burden of late night trips to the local jail, dealing with the police, the courts, the schools, and grieving a death.

- Drug use doesn't mix with school, sports, and the other activities of a teen. Most families do not believe that drug use can be reconciled with the values held by their family. This is a tough time to grow up as a teen. Compared to 25 or 30 years ago, today's teen faces increased risks for all manner of life-threatening situations, whether that be suicide, teen pregnancy, contracting HIV, or being involved in a homicide. At the very least, teens need to know that drug use makes doing well in school harder, that it will affect their emotional life, and that it will make it more difficult to make and keep "quality" friends. Teens today need every break they can get to protect their health and potential for success.

Facing the Problem

One of the grander myths about the American family is that a family solves its own problems, quietly and effectively. A family is strong and supportive—a last sanctuary for any problem or crisis. When it comes to helping a teen stop using drugs, many families try to promote this myth of the American family and hide the problem, or go just the opposite route and find blame for the problem in every aspect of society except their own family and their teen. Getting a teen off drugs and keeping that teen off drugs—regardless of the drug—is tough, grueling, and often-painful work. A family needs to admit and accept their teen's drug use, reserve blame, and

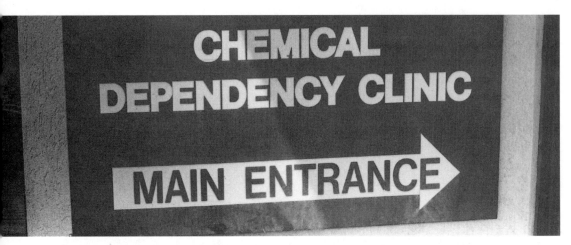

Caring adults may find they need to admit their adolescent to a hospital or drug rehabilitation center. There is absolutely no shame attached to getting help. The shame is if one does not.

look forward with the single, sole-minded task of getting their teen off drugs. Neither dropping a teen off at a hospital or rehabilitation center and hoping for the best, nor denying the problem—simply ignoring the drug use or taking blame for the problem—works. The figures and statistics about recovery from drug or alcohol abuse are grim. Caring adults can either be involved on the upside to recovery or the downside to continued use. These are the same options available for a teen using drugs.

Recognizing the Problem

The first step for families is to recognize that there is a problem. For better or worse, there are any number of objective factors that point toward drug use. For example, traffic tickets for driving under the influence of alcohol are very good indicators of alcohol abuse. Low grades, absenteeism, withdrawal from family activities, unexplained injuries or accidents, substantial behavior changes, or stomach upsets can also be objective indicators of a drug problem. However, those indicators are often more complex than answering a simple question: "Where is my teen spending his or her time, and what is he or she doing during that time?" It takes time to get drugs, use drugs, and then return home. Another simple way to ask the same question is, "Where is my teen spending his or her energy?" The fewer answers you have to the questions above, the more you need to know. It is not normal for a teen to be out all night, sleep during the day, and then be unexpectedly frantic to go out the next night. When you think about drugs and your teen, think objectively and coolly.

Denial

Most people with a drug problem will deny it. Generally, the greater the problem, the greater the denial. For this reason, prying facts about drug use out of teens is usually not very productive. Most people have more success presenting their teen with a list of objective behaviors that point to a problem that they want to solve with their teen. Sometimes the problem is something else. Give your teen a break. Stick to the facts, and ask your teen to respond. If you are uncomfortable with such a confrontation, contact a local crisis center or community health agency and ask what they think about your observations and how you might proceed. There may be an underlying depressive illness causing your teen to seek "self-medication." A crisis center may be able to help you sort out the facts, identify the problem, consider possible solutions, and then decide what to do next.

Alcoholism in Your Family

Let your teen know if there is a history of alcoholism in your family. No amount of shame or pride should keep you from being straightforward about your family history. Many, many young lives would be saved the slow death of alcoholism or pain of recovering from alcohol by knowing at an early age that alcohol may not be something they can handle, even in small amounts, because of a genetic risk in your family.

Your teen needs to know the basic facts about alcohol, facts that other teens usually do not know—facts that special interest groups spend millions to distort and glamorize:

- Alcohol is a drug. Specifically, alcohol is a depressant.
- Alcohol slows body functions, coordination, and the ability to think and react.
- Alcohol affects everyone differently, but, in general, body weight and the amount of alcohol consumed over time are the two most important factors.
- Alcohol affects judgment and lowers inhibitions. Teens who are drinking or drunk do things they would not ordinarily do. Behaviors range from becoming upset emotionally, fighting, using other drugs, participating in unplanned sexual activity, including unsafe sex—to drinking and driving.

Teens should also know that drinking very large amounts of alcohol over a short period of time, say a tumbler full of hard liquor, could cause sudden death. Finally, alcoholic beverages should never be confused with poisonous products that contain alcohol. Rubbing alcohol, for example, is not an alcoholic beverage and may be fatal if swallowed.

As with all discussions regarding drugs, families need to set clear expectations for behavior, clear rules, and clear consequences for breaking the rules, without making drinking seem like something appealing to do because it is forbidden.

Helping Teens Say No to Drugs

There is more involved in preventing drug use than just setting rules. The developing adolescent needs a strong sense of self-esteem, along with the social skills necessary to withstand peer pressure to participate in substance abuse and other risky behaviors. The developing adolescent needs to know that he or she is loved and valued as a person.

Planning and spending time with your adolescent on a daily basis is the key to lasting success. Your young person needs to see how the rules you have set work with the experiences they have outside of the home, at school, or with friends. The consequences of breaking rules are very important. It is also important for him or her to know that you are aware of the drug use in your community and the fact that he or she will be offered drugs and will have the opportunity to use drugs.

Many young lives would be saved the slow death of alcoholism or pain of recovering from alcohol by knowing at an early age that alcohol may not be something they can handle because of genetic risk in your family.

Families need to give their teen every possible, simple way to refuse drugs. You need to be willing to work with your teen on easy, no-nonsense ways to say no to drugs. In most cases, this means putting yourself in the role of the heavy. A teen who says, "I made a deal with my family not to use drugs" faces fewer questions than a teen left facing their peers alone. Likewise, a simple, short answer for saying no to drugs holds up better to follow-up questions. "Look, what can I say, I made a deal with my family," is a simple, straightforward response—one that can be followed by another, equally simple response. "Don't you get it? A deal's a deal, and I'm keeping my end of the bargain."

Adults who expect their teens not to use drugs have to be willing to listen to their teens talk about the pressures to use drugs that are around them. Adults must listen carefully when teens talk about the situation. Parents need to work with their teens to help them resist drugs, and to immediately correct any lapses in the no drug use rule. The more your teen is willing to talk with you about drugs, the better the chances that your teen will stay off drugs.

A GUIDE TO TEEN PARTIES

Parties have been a fact of life for teens and families forever. The right kinds of parties can be an important factor in your teen's growth into adulthood. The planning of a party, and even talking about going to parties, can help build trust between you and your teen. You also need to be aware of your responsibilities—to your teen and to your family—when your son or daughter wants to go to a party or have a party at home.

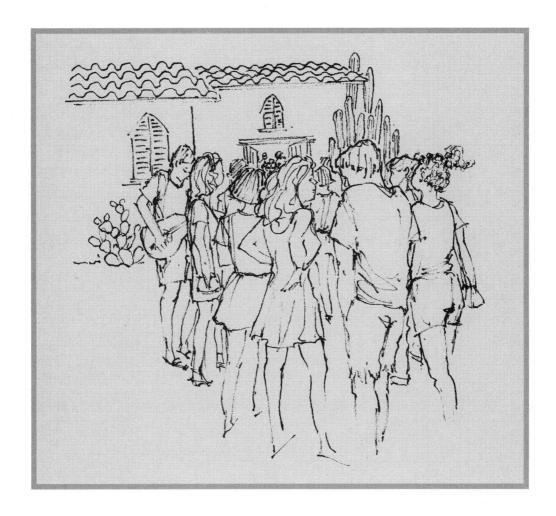

When the Party is at Your House

By high school, teens should be capable of planning a party of their own. Your responsibility is to set the broad guidelines for the party.

- No open houses and no crashing. You need to make sure that your teen understands that unwanted guests are just that—unwanted.
- No smoking, alcohol or drugs.
- House rules apply. Party or no party, your teen needs to know that the standards of conduct you have set for your household apply during a party.
- No wandering around the house or leaving the party and coming back. Teens should not have access to bedrooms or be allowed to be outside in your neighborhood.

You also need to know your own increasing responsibility for parties given in your home. The two largest problems are uninvited guests and the use of alcohol and drugs. Do not put the burden on your teen to be an adult and enforce the ground rules of the party. Your presence needs to be felt. It does not need to be overbearing. Make sure that your teen knows that he or she can come to you for help if the party starts to get out of control.

In some states it is against the law to allow anyone under age 18 to smoke (in your home or otherwise), or to allow anyone under 21 to drink alcohol. Adults are often legally responsible for anything that happens to a minor who has used alcohol or drugs in their home. Check your state laws carefully before agreeing to a party. Penalties can include jail time and fines.

When Your Teen Goes to a Party

There are a few simple rules to follow if your teen wants to go to a party, dance or other social event:

- Know exactly where your teen is going and with whom he or she is going.
- Know that adults will be present. If necessary, call and check.
- Know when the event is to start and when it will be over.
- Know how your teen is getting to and from the event.

When you decide whether or not to let your teen socialize, consider two important factors: How willing is your teen to follow your guidelines? How willing are you to plan in advance with your teen to help him or her avoid or get out of bad situations?

Any rules you set should at least include an agreement to call home if anything unusual comes up. This means that your teen knows that whatever happens—such as needing a ride because a date has been drinking—you will help out. For kids in high school, it is best to allow your teen to save face and agree to meet you a short distance away from the party or event. Make it easy for your teen to choose this option by agreeing not to punish or restrict your teen for whatever it is that has happened. The next morning is the time for serious discussions and reinforcement of the "no use is acceptable" message.

When You Are Away from Home

Unsupervised parties are never a good idea, whether at your home or at someone else's. Your teen needs to know that you forbid parties while you are away because you will be held responsible for events that occur in your absence. Make sure your son or daughter understands that this is not a matter of trust between you. The facts are that you, as a parent, are legally liable to other young people who may get in trouble at your house. Your teen also needs to know the dangers of attending parties where there is no adult supervision. Remind your adolescent of how quickly a bad situation can develop without any adults around.

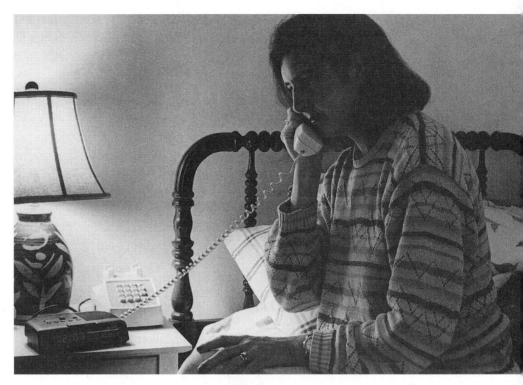

A good rule to have is: "No matter what the hour is, we will come for you if your date has been drinking, or if the party gets out of hand."

Some schools have family member meetings to help set up networking. If you have already had contact with the families of your son's or daughter's classmates, you may feel more comfortable contacting them when a party is planned. Teens also benefit because they know that adults are communicating with each other, and they will thus be less likely to end up at "unauthorized" parties. Your adolescent may not like that you call another parent to see if adults will be present at this party. But your child's safety is a more important concern.

TEENS AND DRIVING

Statistically, teenage drivers are more prone to crashes than any other age group behind the wheel of a car. That said, parents might want to consider these following suggestions before handing over the car keys and allowing your teen to drive.

Remind your teen that driving is a privilege—not a right—and the luxury can be quickly taken away if rules are not strictly followed. Only allow a limited number of occupants in the car when your teen is driving, thus allowing for fewer distractions. Be sure to ask your teen who will be in the car and where they plan to drive. Consider whether they will end up at a destination where drugs or alcohol will be available. Some parents draft a contract with their teens, letting them know that their driving privileges will be revoked if they receive a ticket. It is also a good idea to watch your teen when they pull out of the driveway to make sure that they are wearing their seat belt and paying attention to possible obstacles in the street. Finally, examine the car after they return it. Are there scratches or dents you have not seen before? What about empty beer bottles or other signs of alcohol use in the vehicle?

Following these easy tips could prevent your teen from getting behind the wheel of the car and making a decision that could forever affect his or her life, and the lives of others.

SUBSTANCE ABUSE PREVENTION THROUGH HEALTH EDUCATION

Drug prevention is a team effort requiring cooperation among parents, school officials and community leaders. As parents, you will want to review your school's health education program to be sure of its content. In 1985, for example, parents and community organizers came together to form the Michigan Model for Comprehensive School Health Education. Some central ideas to this successful program are:

- Families are their children's most important health teachers.
- Health education and being well heighten personal and academic success.
- Illegal drug use is wrong and harmful.
- Violence can be stopped through teaching conflict management.
- Good health comes from making wise choices early in life.

Research in drug prevention education has flourished for more than two decades. Unfortunately, the results of this research are usually published in highly technical academic journals, and are not easily available to busy parents and caregivers. Teachers and administrators are focused on the total education of our nation's young people. Now, with the research and publications generated by an organization called "Drug Strategies," concerned citizens and educators have tools for identifying promising prevention curriculum. Drug Strategies is a non-profit organization that promotes effective approaches to the nation's drug problems and supports private and public initiatives that reduce the demand for drugs.

A major publication from this organization, called *Making the Grade: A Guide to School Drug Prevention Programs*, published in 1999, is listed in the references and resources section of this chapter. In addition, APPENDIX 3 in this book presents nine key elements of effective drug prevention curricula, and eight top drug prevention programs in the U.S., as recommended in *Making the Grade*. It is important for parents and caregivers to determine if the drug prevention program being used in their school measures up to the eight top programs. They will want to compare the program their adolescent is receiving with the elements of effective drug curricula. Please bring *Making the Grade* to the attention of school board members, teachers, and administrators.

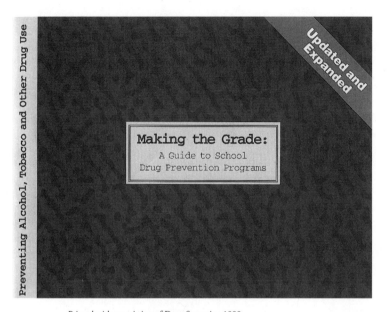

Printed with permission of Drug Strategies, 1999.

REFERENCES & RESOURCES

Adult Children of Alcoholics (ACA): P.O.Box 3216, Torrance CA 90510 USA. 310-534-1815 (message only). Adult Children of Alcoholics is a "Twelve Step" program of women and men who grew up in alcoholic or otherwise dysfunctional homes. The groups meet with each other in a mutually respectful, safe environment and acknowledge their common experiences. They discover how childhood affected them in the past and influences them in the present, and take positive action. E-Mail addresses: info@adultchildren.org (general information, meeting registration) and literature@adultchildren.org (literature orders). Web site: www.adultchildren.org.

Al-Anon/Alateen: Al-Anon Family Group Headquarters, Inc., 1600 Corporate Landing Parkway, Virginia Beach, VA. 23454-5617. General information: 757-563-1600, 757-563-1655 (fax). For meeting information in the U.S. and Canada, 888-4AL-ANON. Al-Anon's primary purpose is to help families and friends of alcoholics recover from the effects of problem drinking. The only requirement for membership is to have a problem of alcoholism in a relative or friend. Alateen is a fellowship of young Al-Anon members, usually teenagers, whose lives have been affected by someone else's drinking. Web site for Al-Anon/Alateen: www.al-anon.org. Web site for Alateen: www.al-onon.org/alateen.html.

Alcoholics Anonymous Worldwide Services: A.A. General Service Office for U.S./Canada: 212-870-3400, 212-870-3003 (fax). 475 Riverside Drive, New York, NY 10015. Alcoholics Anonymous is a fellowship of men and women who share their experience, strength and hope with each other that they may solve their common problem and help others to recover from alcoholism. The only requirement for membership is a desire to stop drinking. There are no dues or fees for AA membership. AA is not allied with any sect, denomination, political group, organization or institution. AA World Services Web site (available in English, Spanish, French): www.aa.org.

Alcohol: Chemistry & Culture, Kevin R. Scheel (Health Educ Pub Co, 1994, $3.95). Outstanding booklet with extremely thorough coverage of all aspects of alcohol consumption including the physical and emotional aspects of use.

American Council on Alcoholism: 800-527-5344, 2522 St. Paul Street, Baltimore, MD 21218. ACA was formed in recognition of the need for a national agency to provide a cohesive, realistic, and coordinated approach to and understanding of the disease of alcoholism. ACA is a forum for addressing the complex issues of prevention, early identification, and treatment of alcoholism, as well as other related alcohol use and abuse issues. ACA believes that most people can use alcohol responsibly. ACA is dedicated to educating the public about the effects of alcohol, alcoholism, and treatment, in the belief that a well-informed public is the best long-term defense against alcohol abuse and alcoholism. E-mail Address: acal@smart.net. Web site: www.aca-usa.org.

Binge, Charles Ferry (Daisyhill Press, 1992, $8.95). This book begins with an 18 year old youth waking up in a hospital minus a foot, following a drinking binge. The story then works to patch together details of his drinking binge, during which he ran over four people with a stolen car before hitting a tree. Ferry shows his main character wheeling, dealing and stealing his way from drink to drink. The book captures the denial, self-deception and consequences of the young alcoholic's life. Note: Read this book before passing it on to your adolescent. Its contents, as explicit as they are and drawn from a life of alcoholism, can save the lives of many young people.

Center for Substance Abuse Prevention (CSAP): 5600 Fishers Lane, Rockwall II, Suite 800, Rockville, MD 20857, 301-443-0365. CSAP's mission is to provide national leadership in the federal effort to prevent alcohol, tobacco, and other drug problems. NCADI is under this program (see listing below). Web site: nnadal@samhsa.gov.

Children of Alcoholics: Selected Readings, Claudia Black, Hover Adger Jr., Steven Wolin, Stephanie Brown, Jerry Moe, et al. (National Association for Children of Alcoholics, 1996, $12.95)). Extraordinary collection by renowned writers and researchers. This monograph represents a variety of perspectives and professional experiences. The contributing writers are among the most distinguished clinicians and researchers in the family addiction field, and here they bring together impeccable research and intuitive clinical experience. The National Association for Children of Alcoholics (NACoA) believes the articles in this book will be useful to those whose interest in the subject is either personal or professional.

The Coaches Playbook Against Drugs (U.S. Department of Justice, Office of Juvenile Justice and Delinquency Prevention, 800-630-8736. 1998, No. NCJ 173393, free). Excellent guide offered by the Justice Clearinghouse, which offers easy access to topics relating to delinquency prevention and juvenile justice.

Coping with Peer Pressure, Leslie S. Kaplan (Hazelden Information Education, 1997, $6.95). Peer pressure strongly influences young people's attitudes and behaviors. Many factors affect how it feels and how a teen will respond to its force. Pressure to use alcohol and other drugs, to become involved in gangs, to have sex, and to wear certain clothes, are discussed by the author. Kaplan's use of vivid personal stories and vignettes make the issues that teens struggle with come alive. Can be directly ordered from Hazelden at 800-257-7800 (item #1158) or from Web site: www.hazelden.org/.

Drinking: A Love Story, Caroline Knapp (Delta, 1997, $11.95). The roots of alcoholism in the life of a brilliant daughter of an upper-class family are explored in this stylistic, literary memoir of drinking by a Massachusetts journalist. The author's personal story of her struggle with alcoholism includes her conclusion that an alcoholic's body responds differently to liquor than a non-alcoholic's body.

Growing Up Drug-Free: A Parent's Guide to Prevention. This publication will help you guide your preschool-to-high school-age children as they form attitudes about drug use. It provides answers to children's questions as well as sources for help. It covers such important topics as: how to carry on a continuing dialogue with your children on the subject of drugs (research has found that although nine out of 10 parents questioned said that in the past year they had talked to their teens about drugs, only two-thirds of the teens agreed); why occasional alcohol, tobacco or other drug use is a serious matter; parent education through providing a working knowledge of common drugs—their effects on the mind and body, the symptoms of their use; the latest drug slang, and methods of drug use now in vogue. The full text of this public domain publication is available at the U.S. Department of Education's Safe and Drug-Free Schools Program home page at http://www.ed.gov/offices/OESE/SDFS. For more information, please contact: U.S. Department of Education, Office of Elementary and Secondary Education, Safe and Drug-Free Schools Program, 400 Maryland Avenue SW, Washington DC 20202-6123, 202-260-3954.

Health Resources Online: A Guide for Mental Health and Addiction Specialists, Laurie Sheerer, Colette Kimball, Steven Ungerleider, Glenn Meyer, and Brian L.P. Zevnik, eds. (Integrated Publishing Inc., 1999, $24.95). Contact to order: Integrated Research Services Inc., 66 Club Rd., Suite 370, Eugene OR 97401, 888-785-6599, 541-683-2621 (fax). E-mail address: lainteg@cerfnet.com. This is an outstanding 300-page resource. Titles, addresses, and reviews of over 300 Web sites, including: newsgroups where you can discuss behavioral health topics, federal government Web sites listed in alphabetical order, state government Web sites listed by state. The book will not only assist professionals in the mental health and addiction fields, but is useful to anyone who needs carefully reviewed information in these areas. Book Web site: www.healthy-resources.com.

Keeping Youth Drug-Free: A Guide for Parents, Grandparents, Elders, Mentors, and Other Caregivers (1996). This booklet provides guidelines to parents and caregivers on communicating with youth about drug prevention and on helping them make positive decisions. Available free from the National Clearinghouse for Alcohol and Drug Information (see organization address below).

Making the Grade: A Guide to School Drug Prevention Programs (Drug Strategies, 1996/1999, $14.95). To order direct: Drug Strategies, 1575 Eye Street NW, Suite 210, Washington DC 20005 or 202-414-6199 (fax). 202-289-9070 for information. This guide is an important tool for identifying promising prevention curricula. It helps teachers, school principals, and concerned citizens determine how to spend scarce prevention dollars. Many parents assume that school prevention programs will protect their children from drugs; *Making the Grade* helps them judge for themselves the adequacy of these efforts. The new *Making the Grade* examines family components of prevention curricula more closely and discusses in greater depth the importance of evaluation and fidelity of implementation. This is a very important publication that reviews 50 school-based drug prevention programs and carefully selects eight to receive top marks. It should be at every school. Parents, caregivers, and administrators will want to be sure it is. See Appendix 3 for a listing of *Making the Grade's* nine key elements of effective drug prevention curricula and the eight top drug prevention programs in the U.S.

Mothers Against Drunk Driving (MADD): 511 East John Carpenter Freeway, Suite 700, Irvington, TX 75062, 214-744-6233 or 800-GET-MADD. This is a non-profit grass roots organization with more than 600 chapters nationwide. MADD is not a crusade against alcohol consumption; the focus is to look for effective solutions to the drunk driving and underage drinking problems, while supporting those who have already experienced the pain of these senseless crimes. It is open to all people, not just mothers. Web site: www.madd.org.

National Association for Children of Alcoholics (NACoA): 888-554-2627 (help line), or 301-468-0985, 301-468-0987 (fax). 11426 Rockville Pike, Suite 100, Rockville MD 20852. NACoA is a national membership organization that advocates and provides educational resources to give support and hope to the over 11 million children under the age of 18 who have an alcohol or other drug addicted parent. E-mail Address: nacoa@charitiesusa.com. Web site: www.health.org/nacoa.

National Association for Native American Children of Alcoholics (NANACoA): PO Box 2708, Seattle WA 98111-2708, 206-903-6574. NANACoA's objectives are: establishment of a national network for Native American children of alcoholics; development of educational and supportive information for Native American communities which include publications, videotapes and posters; conducting annual national conferences for Native American children of alcoholics and others working in Native communities to come together to heal and recharge energies; informing local and national policymakers about the needs of Native American children of alcoholics and influencing positive change toward healthy communities. Web site: www.nanacoa.org.

National Association of Therapeutic Schools and Programs. This association is just getting off the ground as of this writing, and will serve as a review source for the quality of alternative schools designed to help young people who are troubled by depression, drug addictions, difficult family dynamics, abuse or trauma. These alternative schools often combine academic programs with therapeutic programs; many have wilderness learning experience components. John Reddon, the Director of the new association, states that the primary function of the association is to serve professionals and organizations. However, he is very excited about being able to assist parents directly also. The association will have a Web site available in the late fall of 1999, which will serve as a rich source of information specifically for parents, with many links to other relevant information sources. Web site: www.natsap.org.

National Black Alcoholism & Addictions Council (NBAC): 1101 14th Street N.W., Suite 630, Washington, DC 20005. NBAC is a non-profit organization of Black persons concerned about alcoholism and other drugs of abuse. The organization remains the only nationwide, voluntary organization to address the problems and concerns related to alcoholism and other drugs of abuse among Black people. Alcoholism is viewed as the number one health and social problem in the Black community. NBAC is therefore committed to educating the public about the prevention of alcohol abuse, alcoholism, and other drugs of abuse, increasing services for alcoholics and their families, providing quality care and treatment, and developing research models specifically designed for Blacks. Web site: www.borg.com/~nbac.

National Center for Tobacco-Free Kids: 1707 L St. NW Ste. 800, Washington DC 20036, 202-296-5469 or 800-284-KIDS. The Campaign For Tobacco-Free Kids is the country's largest non-government initiative ever launched to protect children from tobacco addiction and exposure to second-hand smoke. The campaign is working to: alter the nation's social, political and economic environment regarding tobacco; change public policies at federal, state and local levels; and increase the number of organizations and individuals involved. This requires actively countering the tobacco industry and its special interests. Web site: www.tobaccofreekids.org.

National Clearinghouse for Alcohol and Drug Information (NCADI): 800-729-6686, 800-487-4889 (TDD). P.O. Box 2345, Rockville, MD 20847-2345. NCADI is the world's largest resource for current information and materials concerning substance abuse. NCADI services include: an information services staff (English, Spanish, TDD capability) equipped to respond to the public's alcohol, tobacco, and drug (ATD) inquiries; the distribution of free or low-cost ATD materials, including fact sheets, brochures, pamphlets, monographs, posters, and video tapes from an inventory of over 1,000 items; and a repertoire of culturally-diverse prevention, intervention, and treatment resources tailored for use by parents, teachers, youth, communities and prevention/treatment professionals. Provides local referral contact information through Regional Alcohol and Drug Awareness Resource Network (RADAR). Web site: www.health.org.

National Coalition of Hispanic Health and Human Services Organizations (COSSMHO): 1501 16th NW, Washington DC 20005, 202-387-5000. COSSMHO is the sole organization focusing on the health, mental health, and human services needs of the diverse Hispanic communities. COSSMHO's membership consists of thousands of front-line health and human services providers and organizations serving Hispanic communities. Web site: www.cossmho.org.

National Cocaine Hotline: 800-COCAINE. Phoenix House, 164 West 74th Street, New York NY 10023, 212-595-5810 x7581. A public service of Phoenix House, 800-COCAINE provides general information regarding substance abuse, and treatment referrals in the caller's area. Treatment options include both inpatient and outpatient programs, and self-help groups. Web site: www.4woman.org/nwhic/references/mdreferrals/nch.htm.

National Council on Alcoholism and Drug Dependence (NCADD): 800-NCA-CALL. NCADD provides education, information, help and hope in the fight against the chronic, often fatal disease of alcoholism and other drug addictions. NCADD is a voluntary health organization with a nationwide network of affiliates. It advocates for prevention, intervention, research and treatment, and is dedicated to ridding the disease of its stigma and its sufferers from their denial and shame. E-mail Address: national@ncadd.org. Web site: www.ncadd.org.

National Drug and Alcohol Referral Hotline: 800-252-6465 24 hours a day. Referral to local AA, Al-Anon, Nar-Anon and Alateen inpatient and outpatient services.

National Inhalant Prevention Coalition: 1201 W. Sixth St., Suite C-200, Austin, TX 78703, 800-269-4237. Offers inhalant resource and prevention materials, as well as treatment referrals for inhalant abusers.

The National Substance Abuse Helpline: 800-378-4435. A 24-hour hotline which provides crisis intervention and gives information and referrals.

Parenting for Prevention, David Wilmes (Johnson Institute, 1989, $15.00). Individual copies free from Miller Family Foundation, Box 831463, Stone Mountain, GA 30083. Parents and other concerned adults who read this book thoughtfully and follow its recommendations will have new insights into a whole host of everyday parenting problems as well as practical skills for handling them.

Partnership for a Drug-Free America: The Partnership for a Drug-Free America is a non-profit coalition of professionals from the communications industry whose mission is to reduce the demand for illegal drugs through media communication. Web site: www.drugfreeamerica.org/ includes extensive drug information, guidance for parents, and further resources. Contact address for donations: 405 Lexington Avenue New York, NY 10174, 212-922-1560.

Playing It Straight: Personal Conversations on Recovery, Transformation and Success, David Dodd (Health Communications, 1996, $12.95). Interviews with celebrities recovering from substance abuse and addiction whose sole purpose is to help others.

Parents' Resource Institute for Drug Education (PRIDE): 3610 DeKalb Technology Parkway, Suite 105, Atlanta, GA 30340, USA, 770-458-9900, 770-458-5030 (fax). PRIDE is a non-profit organization devoted to alcohol, tobacco, and other drug use prevention. E-mail address: prideprc@mindspring.com. Web site: www.prideusa.org.

Safe & Drug-Free Schools Program: U.S. Department of Education, 400 Maryland Ave. SW, Washington DC 20202-6123, 202-260-3954 or 877-433-7827 (public phone: 800-624-0100). The Safe and Drug-Free Schools Program is the federal government's primary vehicle for reducing drug, alcohol and tobacco use, and violence, through education and prevention activities in U.S. schools.

Six Steps to an Emotionally Intelligent Teenager, James Windell (John Wiley & Sons, Inc., 1999, $14.95). A talented psychologist and psychotherapist from the judicial system has written an especially valuable book that is badly needed by many parents and caregivers. He explains how social skills can be developed if adults are consistent in handling discipline, avoid using harsh punishment, set limits, reward acceptable behavior, and seldom use threats or give in to stubborn behavior. Filled with practical help and examples, a must read for adults who want to guide their adolescent toward healthy social relationships.

Students Against Drunk Driving/ Students Against Destructive Decisions (SADD): PO Box 800, Marlboro MA 01752, 508-481-3568. This program was originally developed to encourage students and parents to band together in the fight against drinking and driving, by forming groups that were led by students for students. SADD has decided to incorporate more into its curriculum, and has consequently changed its name to represent all of the situations SADD tries to deal with. Students Against Destructive Decisions is a name that covers the current range of programs, from teen pregnancy to suicide, drug prevention, and gangs. Web site: www.nat-sadd.org.

Straight Talk: A Magazine for Teens (The Learning Partnership, P.O. Box 199, Pleasantville, NY 10570-0199, 914-769-0055, $11.80 for 4-part series). Hard-hitting, to the point publication for teens on HIV/AIDS, self-esteem, substance abuse, and teen relationships. Quantity discounts available for schools.

Terry: My Daughter's Life-and-Death Struggle With Alcoholism, George McGovern (Plume, 1997, $11.95). George McGovern, the 1972 Democratic candidate for President, offers a tragic family drama while confronting the choices of his own life in this story of a daughter's fatal fight with alcoholism. Told in direct prose, the tale is a harrowing one. Teresa Jane McGovern, the middle child of five, began drinking at age 13, was hospitalized for depression after her arrest for smoking pot at age 19, cleaned up for a while in her 30s, but then spiraled out of control until she froze to death in a parking lot after a drinking binge.

Youth Crisis Hotline: 800-HIT-HOME (800-448-4663). A 24 hour crisis line for any crisis for youth ages 17 and younger. E-mail Address: 1800hithome@horizonsd.org.

CHAPTER 8
TEENS AND SEXUAL HARASSMENT

This important chapter draws attention to a pervasive and dangerous practice in schools—sexual harassment. The chapter defines sexual harassment and explains how adults can help the young person who is being harassed. The 1999 Supreme Court ruling related to sexual harassment in schools is briefly detailed. The identified references related to the harassment of gay students are invaluable in assisting families and educators.

HARASSMENT

Your teen may face unwanted sexual attention from another student, a teacher, a coach, or a boss. We used to just ignore this type of behavior, but now we know that sexual harassment is unfair and should not be tolerated. You can help by educating your son or daughter to understand what sexual harassment is. Your teen should also know that she or he should report unwanted sexual attention to you or another trusted adult rather than keeping it a secret. Both girls and boys should be aware of sexual harassment and how to prevent it.

One reason parents give for not talking about sexual harassment with their teens is that they do not understand it. Sexual harassment is unwanted sexual attention at school or at work, and usually takes one or more of the following forms.

- PHYSICAL: Unwanted pinching, brushing against the body, kissing, touching, or rape.
- VERBAL: Sexual or derogatory jokes, comments, or conversations.
- PICTORIAL: Sexual pictures, graffiti, or cartoons.
- SENSORY: Leering, gestures, or whistling.

Although girls are more frequently sexually harassed, teenage boys are vulnerable, too. Here are some examples of harassment of boys and girls:

- Another teen in your daughter's class makes frequent comments about her breast size and asks her whether she's "done it."
- Another student posts a sexual cartoon on your teen's locker.
- Your son's coach suggestively rubs up against him during practice and asks him to stay late to train alone with him.
- Your daughter's teacher tells her that he will give her an "A" if she will make out with him.

Effects of Harassment

Sexual harassment in schools can be a serious problem. One study of students in grades eight to eleven found that 85 percent of girls have experienced sexual harassment, and of those girls, 65 percent were touched, grabbed, or pinched in a sexual way. Another study of teen girls found that 83 percent were touched, pinched, or grabbed, and that 39 percent were sexually harassed at school on a daily basis in the last year. Peer harassment (one student harassing another student) is the most common form of sexual harassment in the schools.

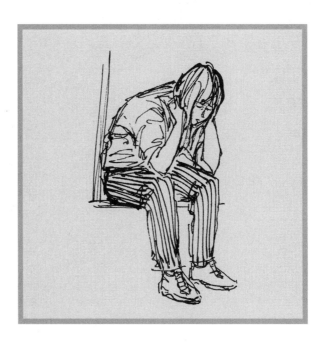

Sexual harassment can have devastating effects on teens. It can cause serious educational, emotional, and physical problems for students and create a barrier to full and equal participation in education. Studies show that 33 percent of girls who were sexually harassed say they do not want to attend school; 32 percent report not wanting to talk as much in class; 28 percent found it harder to pay attention in school; and 18 percent report that it made them think about changing schools. In addition, 64 percent of girls who have been harassed report being embarrassed; 52 percent report feeling self-conscious; 43 percent felt less sure or less confident about themselves; and 30 percent doubted whether they could ever have a happy romantic relationship. Teens suffer even more if their school fails to deal with the problem of sexual harassment.

> Sexual harassment can have devastating effects on teens. It can ... create a barrier to full and equal participation in education.

Some of the most common responses of teens who experience sexual harassment are to deny it to themselves, blame themselves, begin to avoid people and situations, and decide to do nothing. If they decide to do nothing, the harassment often increases. Getting your teen to tell you about being harassed is the first step toward solving the problem.

Support Your Teen

Be open with your teen so that he or she comes to you about sexual harassment. Do not judge how your teen dealt with the harassment. Listen carefully and let your teen know that you are on his or her side. Express your support and that you are proud that he or she told you about the harassment. Encourage your adolescent to create a record of harassment by writing answers to these questions:

- What happened?
- When did it occur?
- Where did it occur?
- Who was the harasser?
- Were there any witnesses?
- What did you say in response to the harassment? (Use exact words if possible.)
- How did the harasser respond to you? (Use exact words if possible.)
- How did you feel about the harassment?

Keep a copy of this record, and then take it to the individual in your teen's school who has been identified as the person who can do something at the school to prevent harassment. Identifying this person is very important if the issue ever needs legal intervention.

Get help for your teen and make sure that the harassment stops. Call your teen's school or place of work where the harassment happened. Take your teen's

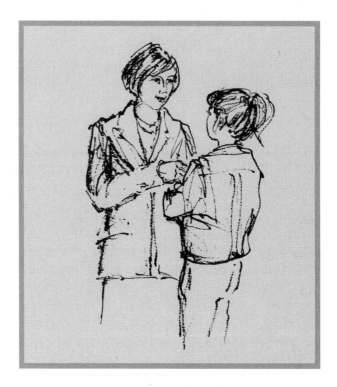

written reports with you. Meet with the principal or company manager to discuss the problem. Request that disciplinary action be taken against the harasser if that is appropriate. Seek professional help for your teen from a source you trust. A counselor or other mental health professional can help you decide what type of help your teen may need. In severe cases, you may want to contact an attorney to discuss your teen's legal rights (see information about 1999 Supreme Court ruling included in this chapter).

Teaching Respect for All

One of your most important roles as a parent is to teach your teen to respect others and to treat them equally and fairly. You serve as a role model for your teen. Your own values, attitudes, and behavior tell your teen how to treat others. To stop sexual harassment before it happens, teach your adolescent respect for women, men, girls, and boys. Show them that it is not right to tell sexual jokes at school or at work. Teach them that no one can touch their bodies without their permission. Help your teen learn the facts about sexual harassment through your actions as well as your words.

EDUCATIONAL POLICY

Prompt and effective attention to the problem of sexual harassment can reduce both its frequency and its devastating effects. Most schools have a policy regarding sexual harassment and a person identified to handle these issues. Work with your teen's school to ensure that all students are protected. A model policy would include the following:

- A clear definition and statement of policy against sexual harassment.
- Programs to educate students and teachers about sexual harassment and the school's policy.
- Information about how to file a complaint.
- A procedure so that complaints are handled in a fair and timely manner.
- A guarantee of confidentiality to the extent possible under the circumstances.
- A promise by the school to act quickly to end sexual harassment and to impose appropriate discipline where necessary.

LEGAL ISSUES

The *New York Times* of March 15, 1997 reports that: "The Office for Civil Rights, which enforces the law forbidding sex discrimination and sexual harassment in schools that receive Federal money, can take legal action against schools that do not have adequate policies to prevent harassment or fail to respond properly to complaints. But what worries schools far more is the threat of private lawsuits brought by parents under Title IX of the Education Amendments of 1972— suits that can lead to damages like the $500,000 that a California jury awarded last fall to a 14-year old girl who had endured months of sexual taunting and threats from a classmate."

"Students must know to go to the principal or other person who can do something about the harassment."

Bruised Bodies, Bruised Spirits: An Assessment of the Current Climate of Safety for Gay, Lesbian and Bisexual Youth in Southeastern Michigan Schools is a report prepared in 1996 by the Gay, Lesbian, and Straight Educational Community of Detroit (GLSEN-Detroit). Based on research, the report focuses on describing and understanding safety and violence as related to sexual orientation from the perspective of school personnel, students, and researchers. This report and *Tackling Gay Issues in School: A Resource Module* need to be in every middle and high school library (see REFERENCES & RESOURCES section for full listings).

Both of these manuscripts serve as an outstanding resource for parents, educators, counselors, and administrators, or for anyone who considers a safe and equitable education to be a right of all students.

The following information has been modified slightly with permission of the ASCD Education Bulletin of June 4, 1999, the biweekly on-line newsletter of the Association for Supervision and Curriculum Development (bulletin@ascd.org).

On May 24, 1999, the U.S. Supreme Court found that public schools might be held financially responsible if those schools are deliberately indifferent to sexual harassment.

But the court decision falls short of being a truly effective tool for stopping sexual harassment, maintains Charol Shakeshaft, a professor at Hofstra University, who has studied peer harassment in schools for more than 10 years. She says, "I'm pleased that the Supreme Court is holding school districts responsible for stopping peer sexual harassment but I think the decision is too restrictive and asks too much."

"For example," Shakeshaft says, "students must make sure they report harassment to the right person. For most students, a teacher is the right person. But not according to the Supreme Court," she observes. "Students must know to go to the principal or other person who can do something about the harassment."

Shakeshaft says that although the ruling extends the rights of those students who are severely sexually abused to claim damages from the school district and administrators, the court sets a very high standard that is not easily met. "In order to receive damages, a harassed student must . . . prove: repeated and pervasive sexual harassment; consistent reporting of this harassment to the correct school official; that the harassment has interfered with the student's grades and learning; and that the school official—upon learning of the sexual harassment—did nothing. "This," Shakeshaft suggests, "is a tall order."

Shakeshaft also takes on those dissenters who fear that the ruling will, in effect, establish a code to regulate behavior that is part of adolescence. She conceded that children have always teased each other and that adolescents experiment with "just how far they can go with the other sex in matters of ridicule, flirtation, and forced physical attention."

"But", she says, "there have been dramatic changes in our social expectations in the past 30 years. Much of what passed for youthful immaturity or childish behavior 30 years ago is very different from what we see today in schools. Sexual harassment," Shakeshaft asserted, "is one of the many ways that students alienate, hurt, and isolate. The Supreme Court ruling which holds educators responsible for stopping sexual harassment is only one incentive for the development of more effective, respectful, and caring adolescent school cultures."

> "Much of what passed for youthful immaturity or childish behavior 30 years ago is very different from what we see today in schools."

REFERENCES AND RESOURCES R/R

Acquaintance Rape. What Is Sexual Harassment? Sexual Harassment. Flirting or Harassment? and *Harassment? Don't Take It!* ETR Associates (P.O. Box 1830, Santa Cruz, CA 95061-1830). For free copies of these five brochures, send stamped self-addressed envelope with 75 cents postage.

"A Blueprint for Action," NOW Legal Defense and Education Fund (99 Hudson Street, New York NY 10013, 212-925-6635). A sheet of tips for preventing sexual harassment at school.

Bruised Bodies, Bruised Spirits, 1996 Report from GLSEN-Detroit. (GLSEN-Detroit, PO Box 893, Birmingham MI 48012. E-mail address: glsendet@aol.com. Detroit has taken steps to assess the current climate of safety in our local schools for gay, lesbian and bisexual youth, with a goal of determining how to assist local schools in creating safe environments for all students regardless of sexual orientation. Includes survey questions and results, policy recommendations for schools, summaries of student stories, and specific examples of anti-harassment policies and report forms.

Everything You Need to Know About Sexual Harassment, Elizabeth Bouchard (Rosen Publishing Group, 1994, $17.95). Focuses on sexual harassment of teens at work.

The Girls' Guide to Life: How to Take Charge of the Issues That Affect You, Catherine Dee (Little Brown & Co., 1997, $14.95). A great resource of ideas, activities, and role models for girls. This book encourages girls to be self-confident and smart, and it gives them guidelines on how to do it! Parents, caregivers, and mentors should add this to the bookshelves of the girls in their lives. Includes photos, illustrations, a timeline of women's history highlights, personal essays by leading women, lists of resources for girls to contact, and more.

Hostile Hallways: The AAUW Survey on Sexual Harassment in America's Schools, American Association of University Women, (AAUW Educational Foundation Research, Dept RR.INT, 1111 Sixteenth St. NW, Washington DC 20036, 202-728-7602, 1993). Represents the first national scientific study of sexual harassment in public schools, finding that 85 percent of girls and 76 percent of boys surveyed have experienced sexual harassment. To purchase, contact the AAUW Sales Office at 800-225-9998 x346. E-mail address: foundation@mail.aauw.org.

Pathways to Tolerance: Student Diversity. (The National Mental Health and Education Center for Children and Families, a public service program of the National Association of School Psychologists). This document addresses the need for an understanding of diversity in our schools and communities. This informative guide for parents, educators, administrators, pupil services providers, and policymakers addresses a broad range of issues and populations. The document provides practical approaches to promote a safe learning environment for children. This document is available free from Victoria Stanhope, NASP, 4340 East West Highway, Suite 402, Bethesda MD 20814. E-mail address: vstanhope@naspweb.org.

Powerplays: A Program for Helping Teens Deal with Sexual Harassment, Harriet Hodgson (Fairview Press, 1993, $8.95). An easy-to-read book that covers all aspects of teen sexual harassment. Explains how teenagers can identify, fight, and prevent sexual harassment in school and on their jobs.

Sexual Harassment: A Question of Power, JoAnn Bren Guernsey (Lerner Publications Co., 1995, $24.00). A look at the latest developments in the way sexual harassment is defined and how harassees have responded, plus suggestions for handling different scenarios.

Tackling Gay Issues in School: A Resource Module, Leif Mitchell, ed., 1998. (GLSEN, 10 Cannon Ridge Drive, Watertown, CT 06795-2445 or call 203-332-1480. E-mail address: glsenct@aol.com. Web site: www.outinct.com/glsen.) GLSEN strives to assure that each member of every school community is valued and respected, regardless of sexual orientation. It is GLSEN's commitment to fight for full inclusion of those who are denied equal opportunity due to oppression based on sexual orientation or gender identity. This book resource grew out of a professional development seminar for the school community. It includes an extensive range of practical information, including: models of anti-discrimination policies, legal facts, curriculum and staff development training activities, administrative strategies for creating safer school environments, information on how to start a student support group, information for parents, and national resources, annotated book resources and Web site listings.

Tune in to Your Rights: A Guide for Teenagers About Turning Off Sexual Harassment, (Programs for Educational Opportunity, 1005 School of Education Building, University of Michigan, Ann Arbor, MI 48109-1259. Call for order form at 734-763-9910 or send your name, address, and a check for $4.00). Defines sexual harassment, identifies warning signals, and provides tips for parents and schools. Includes stories from teens. Program Web site: www.umich.edu/~eqtynet.

"*Working Together to Understand and Stop Sexual Harassment*," (King County Sexual Assault Resource Center, PO Box 300, Renton WA 98057. 206-226-5062). This free booklet features sexual harassment scenarios and dos and don'ts. Send a self-addressed, stamped envelope and specify the booklet's name.

CHAPTER 9
TEEN SAFETY AND CRIME PREVENTION

It may be difficult to face, but the fact is your teen could become the victim of an assault or abuse. This chapter addresses the issues of keeping your adolescent safe, preparing him or her for difficult situations, and knowing what to do if the unthinkable happens.

AWARENESS FIRST

Teens are of the age when they can be away from their families and be more independent—going places with friends or going alone. This newfound freedom becomes a problem for some teens because they feel invulnerable—they take risks. The key to increasing your teen's safety away from home is awareness. The more aware your teen is of possible dangers, the safer he or she will be.

In the teenage years, the desire to belong or fit in is especially strong, which may make your son or daughter go along with unsafe activities or reluctant to leave an unsafe situation. Share the following information with your teen and help him or her understand that being aware is smart, and will help them stay safe.

Statistics show that people who think about possible crime situations and plan what they would do ahead of time are better off. First, they are more aware of their surroundings and therefore are much less likely to be chosen as targets.

Second, they are more likely to be able to keep their wits about them and escape without serious injury if they are attacked.

SEXUAL ASSAULT

Sexual assault is any sexual act committed by one person against another without that person's consent. No matter what it is called—sexual assault, sexual abuse, or date, acquaintance, or stranger rape—such conduct is against the law and is never the survivor's fault.

One state recognizes four degrees of sexual assault, depending on whether the assault consisted of penetration or of contact without penetration, and on the relationship between the assailant and the victim. The legal term for sexual assault in that state is criminal sexual conduct, which puts this crime in its proper perspective and creates a clear-cut distinction between the criminal and the victim.

> Society has long blamed sexual assault on the victim. The facts show an entirely different picture.

Sexual assault is a crime of violence and degradation, and has nothing to do with lust or sex or love, and is never the survivor's fault. Force is a part of any sexual assault, which can be in the form of emotional coercion, implicit threats, verbal threats, or physical force with or without a weapon. Rape is always the responsibility of the rapist, not the person being attacked.

Rape Awareness and Prevention

Few people would say to a victim of armed robbery, "You had it coming." Unfortunately, our society has long blamed sexual assault on the victim. The facts about sexual assault show an entirely different picture.

- One in four women is sexually assaulted before the age of 18.
- One in three women and one in eight men will be sexually assaulted at some time in his or her lifetime.
- Most sexual offenders are someone the targeted person knows and trusts.
- Survivors of sexual assault do not lie about the crime. False reports of sexual assault occur at the same rate as any other crime.

DATING AND SEXUAL ASSAULT

Rape is an unpleasant subject—even more so in dating relationships. We don't want to think about it. We don't want to talk about it. We don't want to believe that this violent crime could happen to us or someone we love. Please review the information below very carefully, and then discuss it thoroughly with your teen.

Help him or her develop an understanding of the facts about date or "acquaintance" rape. Many such crimes go unreported because the survivors feel they somehow invited the attack by going out with the perpetrator. Although this crime is most often committed against women and girls, teenage boys are vulnerable, too (to attack by men or other boys). Most people find it unbelievable, but boys are at great risk because they do not even consider it a possibility, and have no idea what to do. The element of surprise works in the criminal's favor. Young men are also the least likely to report a rape because of the shame involved.

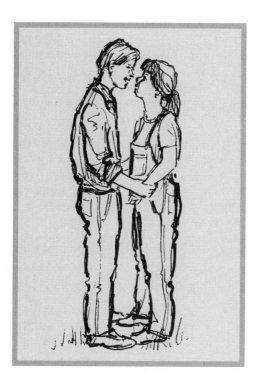

Your teenager needs to know that sexual assault can happen in relationships. Talk with your teen about sexual assault before they start going out with other teens in groups or on dates. Tell your teen that, no matter what the circumstances were that led up to the assault, rape is never his or her fault. Not all rapes can be prevented, but taking some precautions can reduce the risk. Teach your son or daughter these rules.

- Know what your sexual limits and values are. Make sure you have it clear in your mind whether, with whom, and under what circumstances you would engage in sexual behavior, and how much.

- No always means NO. It doesn't matter what the circumstances are, who the person is, or how you feel at the time; no means no. It is never

OK to force yourself on someone. If someone tries to force themselves on you, it is OK to defend yourself.

- Speak up immediately! Silence can be misinterpreted as consent. Communicate to your date your intent and expectations about dating and sexual limits. State your feelings clearly and firmly.

- Stay alert. Drug and alcohol use, besides being illegal, reduce a person's ability to evaluate potentially dangerous situations.

- Act on your gut feelings. Leave an uncomfortable situation—you do not owe anyone anything.

- Do what it takes to stay safe. Scream, yell, or get angry if you must. If people are nearby, yell, "FIRE!" to get their attention. (You may want to practice yelling and screaming).

Self-defense Strategies

There is no single plan or tactic that will work in every assault situation. Your teen needs to know that his or her gut feelings about a situation may be the most important self-defense tool he or she has. Your son, especially, needs to understand that it is possible for him to be sexually assaulted, and that awareness is a means of protecting himself. Discuss these points with your teen.

> Talk to the attacker. Most rapists report that they never considered the victim a person.

- Trust your instincts. If a situation feels unsafe, it probably is. Stay calm, and do not panic—concentrate on your breathing to keep from freezing up. Take your inner feelings seriously and react quickly.

- Get away. If at all possible, get away to somewhere safe and seek help immediately. Never stay in a situation that makes you uncomfortable, whether that is on a date or while walking home alone. Always carry enough money for a phone call and a bus or cab fare home.

- Talk to the attacker. Most rapists report that they never considered the victim a person. Talk about family and parents, or tell the rapist he is hurting you. You may make him see you as more than an object. (Some people have escaped sexual assault by telling the attacker that they have HIV/AIDS or another sexually transmitted disease.)

- Make a scene if other people are nearby. It is perfectly acceptable to shout out loud, "This man is bothering me!" or "Get your damn hands off me!"

- As a last resort: Fight back. Fighting back may stop the assault and create a moment for you to get away, or fighting may increase the intensity of the attack. There is no set rule because every situation is different: Use your best judgment. Statistics do show that survivors who fought back were more likely to stop the attack. If you decide to fight back, no tactic should be attempted halfway—you must use all the strength you have to create a chance to get away.

Don't Give Up

There is no one "right" solution or guarantee in a sexual assault, but survivors who don't give up have a much greater chance of escaping. Not all people are physically or emotionally prepared to defend themselves in an assault. Generally, unless people (this includes adult males) have had a chance to think through and/or practice self-defense tactics, they will be at a disadvantage in a hand-to-hand fight with a criminal.

Self-defense classes may help your teen feel more confident about using a physical response. Ideally, families should advocate for personal protection classes as part of a school's physical education curriculum. Rape crisis programs and community education programs may also have information on self-defense resources.

Detroit News columnist J.B. Dixon, reports the results of a Channel 7 (Detroit) survey of rapists, which revealed that 60 percent would stop an attack if the victim fought back; 63 percent would be stopped by a liquid tear gas or pepper spray, and 67 percent would be stopped by a whistle or alarm.

If Your Teen is Assaulted

Sexual assault is a traumatic and sometimes life-threatening crime. If your teen tells you that she or he has been sexually assaulted, believe him or her, and don't blame your teen for the attack. Your teen is not responsible for the attack—the rapist is responsible.

It is very difficult for a person to share this information. One reason a teen might be reluctant to tell about sexual assault is that teens are often victimized while doing something they aren't supposed to be doing, such as sneaking out of the house, going to a party when they said they were babysitting, or going out with someone they just met at the mall. In that case, it is the lie and fear of getting in trouble that may keep a teen from disclosing a rape (both males and females).

A second very important reason why a person might not want to tell anyone about a sexual assault incident is that the person may be very afraid of retaliation by the attacker. Rapists/sexual predators often threaten the victim with lethal consequences to themselves or loved ones "if they tell." Such a threat can be a very real threat, and is not to be dismissed. Therefore, a teen's silence could be motivated by a desire to protect themselves or others.

Do not let shock, anger, or embarrassment keep you from getting your teen immediate help. You may wish to first call a 24-hour rape crisis hotline for advice on getting help. You can check your Yellow Pages under Crisis Intervention, Hotlines & Helping Lines (after Hotels) or call your hospital or telephone information for a local center. (See REFERENCES AND RESOURCES section following chapter). Most crisis centers have victim assistance programs that will help you get medical assistance, contact the police, and get other professional support. The steps below are recommended in any case of sexual assault.

1. REPORT THE ASSAULT TO THE POLICE IN THE CITY IN WHICH THE CRIME OCCURRED. This step should be taken with your teen's consent as soon as possible after the attack. Talking with the police may be painful for your teen, and for you. Keep in mind, however, that your teen has done nothing wrong and may not be the attacker's only victim.

   If your son or daughter is reluctant to report the crime to police, a rape crisis counselor can help address any questions or fears you or your teen may have about reporting, and may even be able to accompany you to the police station.

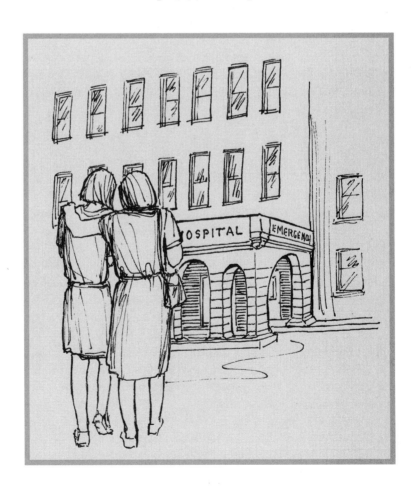

2. SEEK MEDICAL ATTENTION AT A HOSPITAL OR MEDICAL CENTER AS SOON AS POSSIBLE AFTER THE ASSAULT. Medical attention is important for several reasons. First, the exam will help determine if your teen has been physically injured in any way. Second, physical evidence will be collected, which will be preserved for possible prosecution. Avoid letting your teen bathe or shower until after the exam, and bring the clothes that were worn during the assault to the hospital.

The hospital exam will include testing for sexually transmitted diseases. For privacy purposes, you may choose to have HIV/AIDS testing conducted at some other site, such as your County Health Department. If your son or daughter is in an intimate relationship, be sure that you or medical staff discuss the need to practice safe sex pending the outcome of the test results.

The exam will include a pregnancy test if the victim is a woman. If you or your teen have concerns about unwanted pregnancy, discuss this issue with the examiners and ask about the morning after pill.

Most insurance policies will cover the medical exam. If you are uninsured, you may be eligible for crime victim compensation. Your local rape crisis program or Prosecuting Attorney's office can help you file a claim.

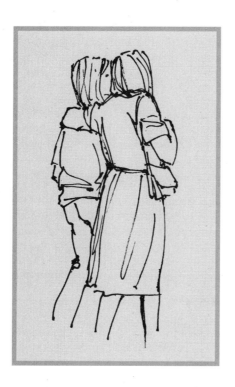

Recovering from an Assault

Your teen needs your love and support after surviving a sexual assault. Fear, depression, anxiety, embarrassment, and feeling powerless are not uncommon among survivors. Your teen may have problems thinking or concentrating. School or work performance may suffer. She or he may become physically ill, be afraid to leave the house, or not want to be touched by anyone. Some teens need professional guidance to work out feelings of anger, shame, and guilt. A counselor from a rape crisis program or a mental health professional can help you decide what kind of help your teen may need.

Family members also suffer after an assault. You may blame yourself for not having protected your teen. You may want to restrict your teen's freedom in the hope that it will prevent further victimization. You may find your teen's behavior toward you is confusing and hurtful. You may fear your teen is "damaged" for life. You need support, too. Talking to a rape crisis counselor or a trusted friend can help you sort out your feelings so that you are better prepared to help your son or daughter recover from sexual assault.

SEXUAL ABUSE

Between 70 and 80 percent of the sexual abuse of young people is by someone they know, trust, or even love. To make matters worse, very few survivors feel able to tell anyone about the abuse. Fear, shame, and confusion often combine to allow the sexual abuse to continue for months and even years. In addition, the attention that the child receives may be filling a void and, therefore, feel satisfying to the child since sexual abuse is usually seductive and not brutish.

> Between 70 and 80 percent of the sexual abuse of young people is by someone they know, trust, or even love.

Parents, family members, and caring adults need to know—and admit to themselves—that sexual abuse can happen to the child or teen they love. The unthinkable can happen. When children are still young, it is important to teach them the concepts of "good" touch and "bad" touch, and to give them a sense that they have a personal space that is not to be violated by anyone. A strong sense of self-worth and personal value enables a child or teen to rebuke this type of overture. In fact, such an overture will probably not be made to a confident child.

Children and teens need to know that they can come to their parents or a caring adult about any situation that makes them feel uncomfortable. You need to understand that sexual abuse is never your child's or teen's fault. You must be prepared to hear that an uncle, a sibling, a teacher, or your spouse is abusing your child, and not blame your child.

Signs of Abuse

Physical signs of sexual abuse may include having sexually transmitted diseases such as gonorrhea or syphilis at a young age. Torn skin in and around the vagina, swelling of the genitals, foul vaginal or anal odor, frequent urination or a painful or burning sensation during urination may also be signs of sexual abuse. Sometimes, pregnancy at age 12 or younger is a sign.

Behavioral signs may include acting in sexually seductive ways or talking about sexual things in a more mature manner than appropriate for the child's age. Some teens may have poor relationships with peers or start fighting at school, or fail to finish school assignments and get low grades.

A teen may also:

- Act pseudo-mature.
- Become depressed.
- Become angry.
- Use drugs and/or alcohol.
- Become self-destructive.
- Have a marked decrease in self-esteem.

The reaction to sexual abuse varies with the individual. It should be noted that some survivors of sexual abuse may react by focusing all of their energy into school work and making the honor roll—becoming the "model" child.

Most victims, however, act out in negative ways. They may run away, have sex with many different individuals (become promiscuous), either think about or attempt suicide, or turn to alcohol and other drug use. A teen may have no friends visit the home, and have problems trusting others. If abused at home, they may spend more time away from home or avoid being around the abuser elsewhere.

A female may become ashamed of her body or develop an eating disorder such as anorexia or bulimia. Girls who have been abused have also been known to mutilate themselves by repeatedly scratching their bodies or biting their lips, nails, fingers, or mouth until they bleed.

Males and females may begin to lie, steal, and get into fights. Despite the lack of correlation, boys may fear becoming homosexual if abused by a male. Boys most often do not tell anyone that they have been abused. Boys also believe they cannot possibly be victims—they must always be brave—and exhibit a macho behavior.

If Your Teen Has Been Abused

Children and teens seldom lie about sexual abuse. Your role is to listen carefully and let your teen know that you are very angry at the abuser and not at your child. Let your teen know that you love him or her. It is important not to ask your teen what role they may have played in the abuse. Don't blame the innocent. Above all, your son or daughter needs to know that you are on his or her side, no matter what.

Getting assistance for your teen and your family is the important next step. Call the police. If your son or daughter has been abused, there are likely to be other victims. Seek professional help from a source you trust. Your doctor, religious institution, or school may be able to provide a referral. Check with your local family service agency, crisis center, or community mental health services agency. Children's Protective Services—listed in the phone book, can also help.

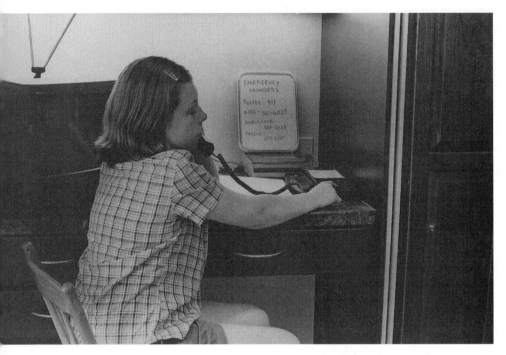

Every teen needs to know how to get help in times of emergency — how to call the police, the fire department, a crisis center, or a trusted friend. Please list the numbers near your phone.

REFERENCES & RESOURCES

Abused Boys: The Neglected Victims of Sexual Abuse, Mic Hunter (Fawcett Books, 1991, $11.00). Written by
a psychologist who has extensive clinical experience treating male victims of child sexual abuse,
this book explodes the myth that sexual abuse of male children is rare, or that the consequences
are less serious than for girls. He examines the physical and emotional impact of abuse on its
victims and the factors affecting recovery. With personal case histories of victims and their
families, this is a powerfully written and meticulously researched book.

Basic Facts About Child Sexual Abuse (National Committee for Prevention of Child Abuse, P.O. Box 94283,
Chicago, IL 60690, 800-835-2671, Order #702480, $4.35) Answers basic questions about abuse.
Also publishes a free catalog.

But What About Me? Marilyn Reynolds (Morning Glory Press, 1996, $8.95). Erica pours more and more
of her heart and soul into helping boyfriend Danny get his life back on track. But the more she
tries to help him, the more she loses sight of her own dreams. It takes a tragic turn of events
to show Erica that she can't "save" Danny, and that she is losing herself in the process of
trying. Finally, Erica is forced to wonder, "But what about me?" She begins the difficult task of
putting her own life back together again. This book puts real-life problems of acquaintance rape
into a candid fictional format that can grab the attention of teen readers the way no amount
of simple lecturing can ever do.

Child Lures Family Guide, Kenneth Wooden (Wooden Publishing House, 5166 Shelburne Road, Shelburne
VT 05482, 802-985-8458, 1996, $5.00). This 4-color booklet offers tips for parents for
protecting kids from molestation and sexual assault. Endorsed by the American Academy
of Pediatrics.

Chimera Self Defense for Women (Chimera Educational Foundation, Inc., 28 East Jackson, Room 1101,
Chicago IL 60601, 312-957-0195). Offers workshops, lectures, and a 12-hour basic self-defense
course for women. Offices located in Georgia, Illinois, New Jersey, North Carolina, Ohio,
Pennsylvania, and Wisconsin.

Citizens Against Crime, Inc. (CAC). CAC is an international company that, since 1980, has specialized
in dynamic personal safety education programs, training, and distribution of high quality safety
products. 800-466-1010. Web site: www.trainingexperience.com.

Keeping Schools & Communities Safe Web Site, (U.S. Department of Education). This is a new Web site
which features publications, funding opportunities, and organizations that can help us keep our
school and communities safe. Web site: www.ed.gov/offices/OESE/SDFS/safeschools.html.

"Love Doesn't Have To Hurt Teens," (American Psychological Association, 750 First Street NE, Washington
DC 20002). In consultation with the Partners in Program Planning in Adolescent Health (PIPPAH).
(The partners are: the American Bar Association's Center on Children and the Law and
Commission on Domestic Violence; American Dietetic Association; American Medical Association;
National Association of Social Workers. PIPPAH is supported by the Office of Adolescent Health
of the National and Children Health Bureau, Health Resources and Services Administration,
U.S. Department of Health and Human Services.) Here is a four-color brochure every family of
teens needs to request for their adolescent. It repeats the information on preventing violence
in teen relationships found in this book so that your teen will read it. It provides perhaps
life-saving hotlines and resources. Web site: www.apa.org.

Streetsmarts: A Teenager's Safety Guide, Jane Goldman (Barron's Juveniles, 1996, $4.95). The author's
commonsense tips generally translate into ways of anticipating and avoiding unnecessary risks
in public places, at school, on dates, at house parties, when using buses and subways, when
traveling at night, and even at home.

The Survivor's Guide: A Guide for Teenage Girls Who Are Survivors of Sexual Abuse, Sharice A. Lee, (Sage
Publications, 1995, $13.95). This short, comprehensive book gives the survivor of sexual abuse
insight into why they feel the way they do. While easy to read, it isn't simpleminded or

condescending. It gives sensible steps that lead toward healing and away from self-destructive behavior. A must read for anyone who worries about how to support survivors.

Teen to Teen: Personal Safety and Sexual Abuse Prevention, Catalina Herrerias (Kidsrights, 10100 Park Cedar Drive, Charlotte, NC 28210. 704-541-0100 or 888-970-5437, 1993, $5.95).

What Are My Rights? 95 Questions and Answers About Teens and the Law, Thomas A. Jacobs (Free Spirit Publishing, 1997, $14.95). Thomas Jacobs, an Arizona Superior Court Judge specializing in family and teen matters, explains the law in easy-to-understand terms. Using a question-and-answer format, the book helps teens see that the laws of the land affect them every day and in virtually every decision they or the adults around them make. By knowing the law—and the consequences of breaking it—teens can recognize their responsibilities as teenage citizens and make informed choices about their future.

What Parents Need to Know About Dating Violence: Learning the Facts and Helping Your Teen, Barrie Levy and Patricia Griggans (Seal Press Feminist Pub, 1995, $12.95). Defines dating violence, demonstrates the warning signs, and explains the psychology of an abusive relationship and how to help.

Chapter 10
Teens and Violence

The issue of violence in relation to adolescents is a difficult yet overwhelmingly important subject to discuss. This chapter addresses, with detailed information and sensitivity, the issues of school violence, domestic violence, abusive teen relationships, media violence, and gang violence.

The Face of Violence

The explosion in juvenile crime arrests that began in the late 1980s has steadily declined over the past several years. Homicide rates among teens between ages 14 and 17 are starting to decline too. At the same time, states across the country are making it easier to prosecute teenagers as adults for violent criminal offenses. Nearly half the states have eliminated a minimal age requirement to prosecute felony crimes. In one state, lawmakers are considering legislation to allow the death penalty for murderers as young as 11.

The United States still has the highest civilian homicide rate of any country in the world. When compared to 21 other developed nations, not only are U.S. homicides staggering in terms of lost human life—some 25,000 Americans are killed each year—the homicide rate for 15-24 year-old males in the U.S. is nearly four times greater than the next nation surveyed.

Children and adolescents are especially affected by violence. Over 2,000 children and adolescents die violent deaths each year. Another 1.5 million children suffer abuse and neglect. To make matters worse, the character of violence involving children and adolescents has changed in recent years.

- More hate crimes are being committed, triggered by the Internet and hidden Web sites that are devoted to racism, anti-Semitism, and other forms of hate.
- Homicide is the most common cause of death in young African-American males and females.
- Handguns are widely available to adolescents. In nearly 60 percent of all teen homicides, a handgun is involved.

Children and teens are becoming violent and committing violent crimes at an earlier age. Huge numbers of first and second graders say they have witnessed violent crimes. The juvenile courts are crowded with murder cases involving 10-year-olds and young adolescents.

SCHOOL VIOLENCE

Amitai Etzioni, University Professor at George Washington University, is perfectly clear in stating the issues that this section will explore briefly to open a broader chapter on teens and violence. Dr. Etzioni says the Columbine High School shoot-

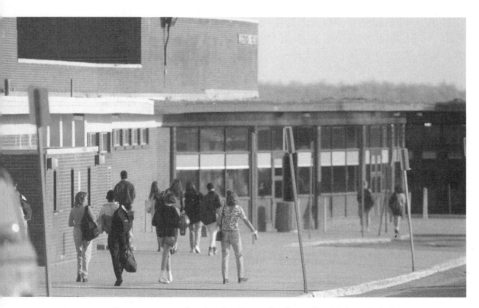

Parents and caregivers need to be deeply involved in school life to help keep schools safe for all.

ings were caused by a combination of several factors, and hence attacking any one of them will not eliminate the problem. He believes there is no silver bullet and no magic cure. But this valid observation should not be used to conceal the fact that guns, the culture, and the Internet each carry some of the blame. It follows that if we tackle any one of these issues, we shall reduce the problem some; if we treat several, we shall do even better. But, truth be told, it cannot be completely licked.

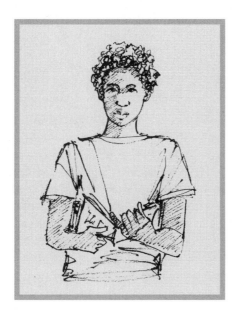

Education

Healthy Teens draws from the philosophy that parents, caregivers, administrators, teachers, and others concerned with youth development can teach children and adolescents self-control and empathy. Lesson after lesson in leading health education curricula use student role play and exercises to teach students how to resist drugs and alcohol, tobacco, and premarital sex. Empathy training begins in kindergarten by teaching youngsters how to identify feelings and continues more in-depth through elementary and middle school lessons. Discussion of important literature and social justice issues also helps to build the character traits of self-control and empathy. Character building modeling by parents, caregivers, teachers, and administrators are of utmost importance. And, as Dr. Etzioni emphasizes: "What schools should help youngsters develop—if schools are going to help lower the likelihood of more Columbines—are two crucial behavior characteristics: the capacity to channel impulses into prosocial outlets, and empathy with others. Teenagers can learn to channel their aroused urges into activities that do not harm others and yet are self-fulfilling. Sports, if properly conducted, provide a major opportunity."

When he discusses sports, Dr. Etzioni refers to sports conducted in the British manner, where it does not matter if you win or lose but how you play the game. While jocks often pick on other students, he says, such behavior is not inherent in athletic activities. Indeed, when any group of students picks on others, or isolates them, this should not be viewed as a reason to cut back on their positive activities, but as an opportunity for education, to develop the much-needed capacity of empathy. Empathy ensures that we will feel the other person's pain, and makes it much less likely that we will hurt, taunt, or isolate that person.

Culture

Hundreds of studies completed at leading universities have come to the conclusion that there is some link between viewing violence on television and in the movies and aggressive acts.

L. Rowell Huesmann, Ph.D., of the University of Michigan, recently told a Senate hearing, "Not every child who watches a lot of violence or plays a lot of violent games will grow to be violent. Other forces must converge, as they did recently in Colorado. But just as every cigarette increases the chance that someday you will get lung cancer, every exposure to violence increases the chances that some day a child will behave more violently than they otherwise would."

> "There has never in the history of the civilized world been a cohort of kids that is so little affected by adult guidance and so attuned to a peer world."

Professor Huesmann has worked on two longitudinal studies related to the effects of television violence. One he is finishing in 1999 has tracked 750 Chicago-area elementary school children for three years.

He indicates, "Boys at age 8 who had been watching more television violence than other boys grew up to be more aggressive than other boys. They also grew up to be more aggressive and violent than you'd expect them to be on the basis of how aggressive they were as 8-year-olds." Professor Huesmann agrees that media violence cannot be singled out as the most important factor in influencing aggressive behavior, but it is one of the pervasive influences.

Manufacturers have produced a variety of software that helps keep certain material on TV out of the view of children and adolescents. These include NetNanny, Cyber Patrol, and the V-chips that are required for new TV purchases. While this software is not a substitute for youngsters learning how to evaluate the media they are viewing or family supervision, it can provide some peace of mind.

The Internet

William Damon, a professor of education and Director of the Stanford University Center on Adolescence, is quoted in the *New York Times* as saying, "There has never in the history of the civilized world been a cohort of kids that is so little affected by adult guidance and so attuned to a peer world. We have removed grown-up wisdom and allowed them to drift into a self-constructed, highly relativistic world of friendship and peers." Damon said that he was stunned when he went to Littleton, Colorado, after the high school shootings there, to find people saying they thought they had no business learning what children were doing on the Internet. The two students who carried out the carnage had vented their hatred on the Internet. Damon said the fact that modern adults have a less black-and-white view of morality and human behavior seems to be blocking their ability to give clear-cut guidance and make strict rules for their children.

New York Times article reissued June 3, 1999 *Detroit Free Press*, p. 3E, with permission William Damon.

Guns

Writing in the *New York Times* of May 26, 1999, Peter S. Bearman, Director of the Institute for Social and Economic Research and Theory at Columbia University, has this to say: "In 1995, roughly 9 percent of all adolescents interviewed in the National Longitudinal Study of Adolescent Health (Add Health Study) once brought a weapon, such as a knife, gun, bat, or club, to school." He indicates that, "In our representative sample of 146 schools nationwide, two-thirds of schools had guns in them on at least one of the 30 days in the previous month." The lesson: Guns are not clustered in a few problem schools. Twenty-five percent of all adolescents report having easy access to guns in their home. Ninety-nine percent of all students attend schools in which at least one adolescent has "easy access to a gun." Dr. Bearman says troubled adolescents with guns are dangerous to themselves and others.

Dr. Etzioni, quoted previously, points out an issue that is a common example of confused thinking about guns. He says, "First, there is no 'right to bear arms' that the press so often speaks of. The Second Amendment to the U.S. Constitution reads, 'A well regulated Militia, being necessary to the security of a free State, the right of the people to keep and bear Arms, shall not be infringed.' The meaning of this right has been tested before the highest court in the land five times over the past 155 years. In each and every case, the U.S. Supreme Court ruled that there are no Constitutional impediments to imposing gun controls on individuals. This is the reason the National Rifle Association (NRA) as a rule does not challenge gun control measures in courts, but instead makes large campaign contributions to legislators, in order to block gun control legislation or repeal it."

Dr. Etzioni indicates that the NRA is right that the diluted Brady Bill, and other such measures, will not do much good. The reason is that the measures are very limited in scope and gun sellers get around them through loopholes larger than ocean liners. Dr. Etzioni states that: "Our children's safety requires not fewer gun controls, but more, of the sweeping and encompassing kind that Canada, Britain, France, and Germany have." As this book goes to print in October 1999, perhaps leadership in state legislatures will provide gun control measures necessary to protect the safety of children and adolescents.

School Violence: What Parents and Caregivers Can Do

There are two important booklets that every school administrator and parent of teens should review. The first resource is *Early Warning, Timely Response: A Guide to Safe Schools,* from the U.S. Departments of Education and Justice (see REF-ERENCES AND RESOURCES section). This carefully crafted booklet outlines exactly what schools need to do to keep students safe, as well as early warning signs of a troubled child. The second resource is the U.S. Department of Education's 1998 Annual Report on School Safety (see REFERENCES AND RESOURCES section). Richard Riley, current Secretary of Education, indicates that the 1998 report describes steps for developing and implementing a comprehensive school safety plan. The report also provides information on what schools, students, parents, business leaders, law enforcement and juvenile justice agencies, and elected officials and government agencies can do to contribute to the creation of safer schools.

Schools cannot be expected to solve all the problems of society; school violence is one of these problems. Many parents and community leaders are already deeply involved in working with their school system to reduce school crime and violence. Please join in this effort—an effort to maintain a safe environment not only for your own children, but for all children in your community.

VIOLENCE AT HOME

Underlying all of the statistics and tragedy of violence in the United States is a single, long-standing truth: The single greatest predictor of future violence is a previous history of violence. In other words, violence begins where children first learn—in the home. This single truth makes domestic violence a matter of public health at the very least, and a matter of national concern if Americans want to break the cycle of violence.

What Is Domestic Violence?

To most people, domestic violence is a husband hitting a wife, or a drunken boyfriend slapping around his girlfriend in the middle of the night. Such simple stereotypes distort what is really behind domestic violence: One person's need for power and control in a relationship. The force can be physical, sexual, or emotional/psychological behavior.

One legal definition of domestic violence is: An assault upon the victim who is the abuser's spouse, former spouse, or a person residing or having resided in the same household, or a person having a child in common with the abuser. The following are a few examples of the many forms domestic violence can take, including forms *not* covered by the laws:

- Hitting, slapping, biting, or burning one's partner.
- Causing injuries such as bruises, black eyes, broken bones, or broken teeth.

- Holding, tying down, or restraining one's partner against his or her will.
- Using a weapon to threaten or injure one's partner.
- Threatening to injure or kill one's partner or the partner's children, family members, friends or pets.
- Forcing one's partner to have sex or engage in unwanted sexual activities.
- Destroying household or personal belongings, and/or hurting or killing pets.
- Preventing one's partner from seeing family members or friends, getting a job, or going to school.
- Keeping all the family money under one's control, and/or refusing to buy food and/or necessities or pay bills.

Animal Cruelty and Domestic Violence

A growing indicator of domestic violence is animal cruelty. Animal welfare agencies and social services agencies say it's a common pattern for a person to abuse or torture animals before committing an act of violence against another person. A recent study at a shelter for battered victims indicated that 71 percent of the women who owned pets reported threats against them, and 58 percent reported actual harm. A Utah State University study shows that pets are 15 times more likely to be harmed or killed in households with domestic violence. Experts say a person who tortures or kills animals is four times as likely to commit a violent act against another person.

How Teens Are Affected

If there is abuse between adults or between adults and children in the home, that abuse permeates the living environment of the child or teen. This environment sets the standards that teens incorporate into their social interactions and dating relationships. These patterns often repeat themselves in the families of the future. Domestic violence, and the resolution of conflict through aggression and violence, leaves the teen with emotional scars that may take years to heal, and may require counseling.

Domestic violence affects people of every age and sex—every ethnic and socioeconomic group. Typically, however, the vast majority of these victims are women. In fact, domestic violence is the largest cause of injury to women between the ages of 15-44 in the United States. The abusers are almost always men. Children and teens living in a home where the mother is abused are more likely to be abused or neglected by the abuser. Those who witness abuse are victims as well. The effect of domestic violence on emotional health is significant.

> Domestic violence is the largest cause of injury to women between the ages of 15-44 in the United States.

What Families Can Do

Parents need to teach their teens positive ways to handle negative emotions—anger, jealousy, sadness—and how to manage their reactions to disappointment, rejection, ridicule, peer pressure, exclusion and conflict.

- Help teens channel or diffuse anger and other negative emotions. Teens need to understand that violence begets violence.
- Learn how to discipline your child without hitting or resorting to verbal attacks (see references listed after Chapter One). The use of verbal and physical abuse at home teaches that this is the way to resolve problems. Kids learn that they can control others by being abusive.
- Control access to television programs. Children and teens are vulnerable to violence and its effects. Violent movies and television shows also seem more real if the neighborhood is filled with assault or homicide.
- Limit access to guns. If your family has a gun, keep it unloaded and in a locked place. Teens and children should not be told the lock's combination or the location of the key.
- Avoid drugs and alcohol. Both substances lower inhibitions and the ability to cope with conflicts. Adults are key role models.

TEEN RELATIONSHIP VIOLENCE

More and more, today's teens are finding themselves in the kind of abusive relationships that in the past have been associated with adulthood, and usually within marriage. The following three sections explain what every adult should understand about teens and the characteristics of abusive relationships. Violence in any relationship is never the tip of the iceberg. Violence is the iceberg, and any proof or sign of violence in your teen's relationship should mean an end to that relationship, whatever it takes to accomplish that.

> The danger in stormy relationships is that the level of violence may increase with each succeeding cycle.

Adults need to clearly communicate displeasure about the violence in the relationship instead of just saying they dislike the teen's friend. Your direct verbal attack on an abuser may make your teen defensive, and make him or her want to stay in the relationship because you disapprove.

Adults need to step in—and step in strongly—in any instance where they believe their teen is being verbally or physically abused, coerced for sex, or has become involved with another teen or young adult that is breaking the law, using drugs or alcohol, or driving drunk.

Abusive Teen Relationship Dynamics

Abusive relationships are not always physically violent. Many times the abuse/violence takes the form of verbal, emotional and sexual behavior designed to intimidate and control the victim. Many men who exhibit increasingly abusive behavior in a relationship are often described as having been very charming and charismatic in the beginning stages of the relationship. It is not always easy to see that violent behaviors are to follow.

As in adult relationships, males are most frequently the abuser. Families of teenage girls should be wary of boys that seem violent, excessively jealous, or show signs of abusing alcohol or drugs. That much is just common sense. You may notice behavior in other young men that simply doesn't make your daughter feel good about herself. You may need to be very direct and ask your daughter what it is that makes a person attracted to someone who makes them feel bad. Below are some of the early warning signs of an abusive relationship.

- ISOLATION: Families and teens need to know that isolation—from other social activities, friends, and even family—is really the first step into an abusive relationship. The abuser seeks control, and there is no better route to control than cutting someone off from all the other things in life that would point to the fact that something is wrong with the relationship. Isolation keeps the victims of abuse silent and allows the relationship to continue.

- FEAR: Intimidation is another key part of abusive relationships. A victim may be subjected to almost constant criticism and made to feel accountable to the abuser for every action. The abuser may be threatening the safety of the victim or other loved ones, or threatening to abandon her.

- BRUISES OR INJURIES: As a caring adult, you have the right to ask your teen about bruises or injuries that you see. You may not get a straight answer back, which in itself should tell you something. Your teen also may try to hide bruises with clothing—long sleeves, slacks or turtlenecks—or sunglasses or excessive make-up. He or she may try to avoid being seen by you for several days after an abusive incident.

Although not always physically violent, pay special attention if your son or daughter is involved in a relationship that is frequently "stormy." The classic pattern for a battering relationship involves cycles of tension and emotional or physical "explosion," followed by apologies and attempts to win the partner back. The danger in stormy relationships is that the level of violence may increase with each succeeding cycle.

Getting Your Teen Out

The victims of abuse are usually the last to see the abuse and frequently the least able to stop the abuse. Abusers are unhealthy people who are unable or unwilling

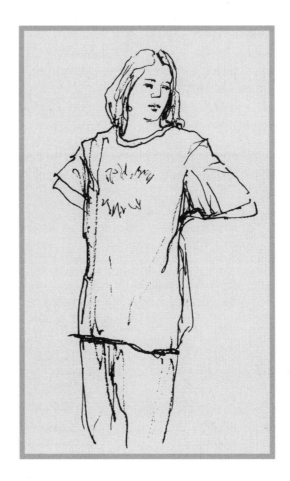

to see the relationship rationally. Your role as a parent is to put an end to the relationship and to protect your teen. Victims of abuse are often reluctant to seek outside help for themselves (or their children). If your teen is a victim of abuse, the first step is to teach him or her to tell someone—you or another trusted adult, a friend, a relative—anyone your teen believes will not blame him or her for the abuse.

If the abuser follows your teen, makes threatening phone calls, or engages in other forms of harassment, you have many practical and legal options. It is important to get expert advice as quickly and reliably as possible. Too often, people without expert training and experience minimize or underestimate the level of danger of the abusive person. Nationwide toll-free hotlines will provide immediately helpful information, such where to find to safe shelters in your community, and what is the role served by personal protection orders (see REFERENCES AND RESOURCES section). If your teen is in danger, call 911.

To end an abusive relationship you may also need to seek help for yourself. Talking with another adult you trust is always a good first step—your religious leader, your teen's counselor or school official, a crisis center counselor or someone in your state or county health department. These individuals may be able to provide referrals for long-term assistance. Again, it is important to link up with someone who already has training and experience with these exact issues. The situation is too complex and too dangerous to handle alone.

There is a national trend toward a decline in reporting abusive relationships or sexual assaults. Much of it has to do with society's habit of placing blame on the victim. In a University of Michigan study, nearly 40 percent of the female participants said they experienced some type of violence in a relationship—yet only 3 percent reported it to the police, and only one-third told anyone.

Many victims are afraid to talk about any abuse or violence that has been done to them or that is currently being done to them. There are many reasons why victims are afraid to speak out. Many times the perpetrator will show much regret over a violent act, and will make promises never to do it again. Unfortunately, the data shows that there is no such thing as a singular act of violence in an intimate relationship. The violence will be repeated, and chances are it will escalate. Another reason the victim may not seek help is because abusive/battering behavior is experienced as trauma, and humans often cannot think straight during or after trauma. A third reason victims can be afraid to talk is because the perpetrator often makes threatening statements that endanger the safety of the victim or the victim's loved ones. The victim might be silent as an act of protection for herself or others.

> Outside consultants are a vital link to helping those involved understand that abusive relationships are a widespread problem and that they are a crime.

A further reason why victims might be afraid to speak out is because they fear a lack of support from family or friends. Although education and the laws about relational violence are changing, there is still much shame involved; many individuals and families falsely believe that these experiences are only happening to them and that the victim is somehow to blame. Outside consultants are a vital link to helping those involved understand that this is a widespread problem and that it is a crime. Domestic violence laws passed in recent years make it much easier to prosecute and convict an abuser. Parents want to show their teen support, patience and understanding when discussing relationship issues.

Choose a comfortable setting when talking to your teen. In that same sense, don't overreact if your teen starts asking questions or expressing opinions. Otherwise your teen will be reluctant to share other parts of his or her life. Teens have a natural tendency to blame themselves when a relationship develops problems. Parents will want to tell their teen that police will treat abusive relationships as a crime, and that you or your teen can report abuse at any time.

As a final note related to getting your teen out of an abusive relationship safely, it is important to know that ending a relationship with an abusive person often does not end the abusive behavior. The findings of a recent research study of battering behavior in marriages are documented in the book, *When Men Batter Women: New Insights Into Ending Abusive Relationships* (See REFERENCES AND RESOURCES section). This information can be used as an index for measuring the risks involved in any battering relationship:

> *We have also learned that the process of escape is fraught with risk. There is no way to know just how risky that process will be in advance. At times, women in our sample were terrified of leaving, but the act of leaving did not lead to continued or increased abuse. At other times, the abuse did continue even after the woman left, and for a period of time became worse. Batterers often become stalkers and escalate their levels of emotional and physical abuse. In the worst-case scenario, homicides occur. Women and children are killed, some batterers kill themselves and their partners, and at times women have to flee their homes, leave town, change their name and identity, and are still found and murdered.*

To the Families of Young Men

Parents and other caring adults, schools, and law enforcement agencies are increasingly holding young men accountable for aggressive behavior or violent behavior that in years past was largely considered "normal." Many families today are teaching their young children and their teens that violence is never the solution to a problem. If you suspect that your son is the abuser in a relationship, understand

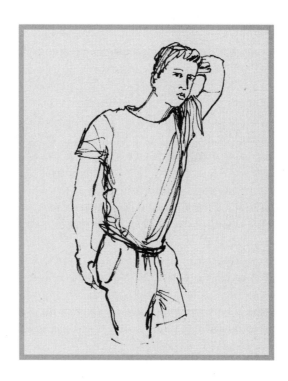

that your son needs help. The first step is putting an end to the abusive relationship. The second step is getting him some professional help.

MEDIA VIOLENCE

From the millions and millions of words spoken and written about violence on television, adults need to know a single, indisputable fact: Overexposure to TV and movie violence has been linked to an increased likelihood of aggression and violence in children and teens. Violence on television is closely linked to violence and aggression in the home, at school, and on the street. Watching violence on television affects how teens view the real world, and how they respond to violence in the real world. Teens who watch a great deal of violence on television come to see the world around them as more violent than it really is. In turn, their worldview is more fearful than necessary. Such teens are more likely to see themselves as the victim of violence. Ironically, this TV-inspired world view leads to a more callused view of real violence, whether shown as indifference to violence against others in general or an unwillingness to take action on behalf of the victim of violence in a specific incident.

> Violence on television is closely linked to violence and aggression in the home, at school, and on the street.

Likewise, violence in video games is linked to violent behavior. Nearly all research indicates that the more violent the video game, the greater hostility and anxiety it produces. Like violence on television, video games tend to reinforce the message that aggression is a part of everyday life. Video games do not enhance hand-eye coordination and they are not a substitute for healthy activity. Some studies even suggest that male teenagers can develop an "addiction" toward playing video games. More important, time spent playing video games means time away from positive activities.

Researchers are still studying the connection between violent lyrics in music and violent behavior. Rap music is heavily criticized for its graphic images of violence, but it also contains more anti-drug messages than any other music style. At the same time, research shows that teens who frequently listen to heavy metal music are more likely to be depressed or susceptible to drugs or alcohol.

Music will always reflect a rebellious attitude in teenagers. It's up to parents to monitor song lyrics and decide if they're suitable for your teen.

GANGS AND VIOLENCE

The police define a gang as two or more people who form an allegiance for a criminal purpose. The gang claims a geographical territory, regularly meets for criminal purposes, and uses intimidation and violence as means for criminal activity. As parents and community leaders, you need information that will help stop gangs from spreading to your neighborhood. You need to understand why teens join gangs, how to recognize gang graffiti and clothing, and most important, how to keep your teen from joining a gang.

Drug Gangs Versus Street Gangs

Police distinguish between drug gangs and street gangs. Drug gangs are concerned only with dealing narcotics and defending their territory. They are smaller than street gangs and are organized with a clear hierarchy, or chain of command. Street gangs are more loosely based and engage in a variety of crimes, from narcotics to neighborhood break-ins. There is no apparent purpose to a street gang, other than to defend its territory.

Communities must identify which gang is on its streets before it can create effective solutions. Is it a drug gang with members from other cities who want to expand their territory? Or a street gang made up of neighborhood teenagers? Law enforcement officials, schools, residents, probation officers, and neighborhood youths can provide data.

Why Teens Join

Boredom, peer pressure, and not enough family involvement are three main reasons why teenagers join street gangs.

Finding legitimate means of earning money is one way to keep teens from joining a gang. Encourage your teen to volunteer, or participate in sports, music or other after-school activities. Take some time to help your child discover what he or she likes to do. Most important, make sure to develop open lines of communication.

> Boredom, peer pressure, and not enough family involvement are three main reasons why teenagers join street gangs.

If your teen has a good sense of self-esteem and feels a part of the family, he or she is much less likely to join a neighborhood street gang. Breaking up a drug gang, on the other hand, will require more traditional means of suppression with assistance from your local police agency and other community groups.

Gangs on the Move

A recent National Youth Gang Survey mailed to 4,120 police agencies indicates youth gangs operate in all 50 states. Many gangs seek to expand their territory by moving from large cities to the suburbs. In some cases, a gang member will "test the waters" in a new area to see if there's a market for illegal narcotics or other gang activity.

Gang involvement also ranges from "wannabes" to hard-core members. Many youths pose as wannabe members without actually joining a gang. But police say a group of wannabes can pose the same threat to a community as a real gang. They don't distinguish between the two groups.

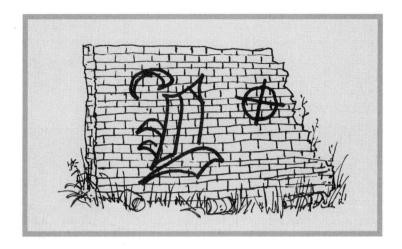

What Is Gang Graffiti?

Graffiti is the inscription or drawing upon walls or other public surfaces. It is a form of vandalism classified by police as "malicious destruction of property." Gangs use graffiti to communicate. Graffiti marks gang territory, advertises the status or power of a gang, warns outsiders away from the gang's territory, and identifies individual members of a gang.

Graffiti places an economic burden both on businesses and homeowners by reducing property values. Area residents learn to fear new graffiti as a sign of potential violence in the neighborhood.

Gang graffiti can be identified by noting the symbols used. A heart, crown, pointed stars, sword, devil's horn, tail, or pitchfork are all commonly used as gang symbols. Symbols that are upside down, crossed out, or split in half are signs of disrespect or a challenge from one gang to another. The misuse of a gang's graffiti is considered very serious and can lead to violent retribution. The letter "K" following the initials of a gang member or an "X" crossing out a gang member's initials are usually a sign of violence, including homicide.

Adults should note that gang graffiti is not always found in public. Gang members, especially younger children not yet in a gang, often draw graffiti on their clothes, books, and papers from school. Gang members show their gang allegiance in a variety of ways. Some gang members identify themselves by tilting their caps to the right or to the left or by wearing bandanas of a certain color or pattern.

Other forms of showing gang ties include the placement of jewelry, the rolling of pant legs, or wearing a certain color of shoelaces. Haircuts, streaked hair, or hair worn with certain rubber bands or barrettes is another sign of gang affiliation. Some gangs alter athletic wear to match gang colors or modify the logos of brand name athletic shoes to match gang logos.

Police officers report that some young teen gang members do not dress in gang clothing or exhibit conspicuous gang behavior. Officers urge continual monitoring of teen behavior and keeping communication links between you and your teen open.

Gangs: What Families Can Do

Teens join gangs to fill a void in their lives, to find things that are missing at home, in school, or in the community. The strongest reason teens give for joining a gang is "wanting to belong." Make sure your teen understands how strongly you feel about gangs:

- Stress the negative aspects of gangs. Point out the negative influences gangs have on individual gang members, families, neighborhoods and the larger community. Focus on the crime, violence, and possible time in jail or prison that gang members face.
- Follow up with your teen if you see any gang graffiti or gang clothing in your home. Let your teen know how much and why you disapprove of gangs, gang graffiti, or gang clothing.

Suggestions to help your teen "belong" to more positive groups

- Know your teen's friends and who influences your teen.
- Know where your teen is and what he or she is doing.
- Help your teen plan constructive days and weekends. Plan family activities, especially activities where you can spend some time alone with your son or daughter.
- Encourage high academic standards, provide reading materials, and discourage excessive television viewing.
- Encourage your teen to participate in school activities.
- Volunteer at your teen's school, whether in a classroom, on a decision-making or policy board, or helping out with extra-curricular activities.
- Form a personal relationship with at least one person at your teen's high school. The person you choose should have the same goals for your teen as you do.

Forming a community coalition is another way to combat gang activity. Coalitions offer teens a way to participate in the community. Coalition members should include parents and students, school and city officials, police, and business leaders. A coalition can help teens develop positive work ethics, and provide volunteer activities, sports, and after-school projects. For example, coalitions can participate in "paint-out projects" to erase graffiti from buildings and overpasses. They can organize Neighborhood Watch programs and offer victim assistance programs.

Parents can start a coalition by registering their group and finding a suitable place to meet. The local high school auditorium or school board office is a great setting for coalition meetings. Federal funding is often available to help purchase office supplies and other material. The National Youth Gang Center assists communities in forming coalitions and developing strategies to combat gang activity. The U.S. Department of Justice can also be contacted about gang violence (See REFERENCES AND RESOURCES section for more information).

If you live in an area affected by gang activity and violence, do not give up. Communities working together and asking for help from business, agencies, religious organizations, and schools can offer alternatives to gang involvement.

REFERENCES AND RESOURCES R/R

Center to Prevent Handgun Violence, (1225 Eye Street NW, Suite 1100, Washington DC 20005, 202-289-7319). Offers information and publications. *STOP I* Brochure/kit available to the medical community. *STOP II* Brochure/kit available to the public. Information to keep your family safe from firearm injury, from the American Academy of Pediatrics. Kits are free, and include posters, six brochures. Sets of brochures available at $15.00 per 100. Web site offers extensive information on firearm safety and archiving of related news items. Special section on kids and guns. Web site: www.cphv.org.

Children of the Night Hotline: 800-551-1300, English and Spanish, (14530 Sylvan Street, Van Nuys CA 91411). This is a privately funded non-profit organization established in 1979. It has rescued over 10,000 boys and girls from prostitution and pornography. Over 80% of these children have stayed off the street and are not dependent on criminal activity. In response to an increasing number of calls from all over the country, the *Children of the Night* hotline became a national hotline. Over 30,000 children call each year to be rescued from pimps, pornographers, drug overdoses, and assaults, which occur on the streets. Too embarrassed to call home, too scared to call the police, *Children of the Night* is often the only resource for teenagers on the street. E-mail address: cotnll@aol.com. Web site: www.childrenofthenight.org.

Children's Safety Network (CSN): National Injury and Violence Prevention Resource Center, (Education Development Center, Inc., 55 Chapel Street, Newton MA 02458-1060, 617-969-7101 x2207, fax: 617-244-3436). CSN provides resources and technical assistance to maternal and child health agencies and other organizations seeking to reduce unintentional injuries and violence to children and adolescents. CSN is one of four Children's Safety Network Resource Centers funded by the Maternal and Child Health Bureau of the U. S. Department of Health and Human Services. Free brochure entitled *Firearm Facts* gives firearm facts on youth suicide and guns, crime, and preventing injuries. Web site gives extensive information, resources, and on line ordering. E-mail Address: CSN@edc.org. Web site: www.edc.org/HHD/csn.

Covenant House's Nineline: 800-999-9999. Children facing crisis situations often find Covenant House by calling the Nineline, a nationwide, toll-free telephone crisis counseling hotline. Trained counselors are available 24 hours a day to provide guidance and support to children and parents, and have access to a database of over 25,000 referral sources. Callers are connected with Covenant House or social service agencies that can best assist them.

Domestic Violence: What Some Women Live With is a Crime, Aimee Argel (State of Michigan Department of Civil Rights, 1995, free). Brochure defines domestic violence, the laws, what people can do to stop the cycle of violence. This brochure can be ordered by calling the "No Abuse Line" at 800-996-6228, which provides emergency and informational assistance for domestic violence, elder abuse, and child abuse. Many other free brochures are available through this line also, including information on how to fill out a Personal Protection Order.

Don't Be the Next Victim: 50 Ways to Protect Yourself Against Crime, Richard W. Eaves and Steven E. Watson (Guardian Press, 1993, $4.95). Paperback packed with common sense, easy-to-follow tips on how to avoid crime.

Early Warning, Timely Response: A Guide to Safe Schools, U.S. Departments of Education and Justice. (U.S. Dept of Education, Special Education and Rehabilitative Services, Room 3131 Mary E. Switzer Building, Washington DC 20202-2524, 202-205-9043, 202-205-5465-TDD, 800-877-8339 or e-mail to David_Summers@ed.gov). This carefully crafted 32-page booklet should be in every school and every home where there are children and adolescents attending school. The booklet outlines exactly what schools need to do to keep students safe, supplemented by a toolkit being released in the fall of 1999, as well as early warning signs of a troubled child (pp. 6-12). Explains how the school needs to act in getting help for troubled children. Its tips for parents are a compilation of statements that are reinforced in detail throughout *Healthy Teens*. Especially helpful and not found elsewhere, is a brief, but excellent section: *Action Steps for Students*. In encouraging students to help create safe schools, parents and caregivers can act as mentors. The *Guide* project was lead by Kevin P. Dwyer, National Association of School Psychologists and David Osher, Project Director American Institute of Research. It was reviewed by an expert panel, followed by a panel of family members, teachers, principals, young people, and major national associations. The full text of this public domain publication is available at the Department of Education's home page at www.ed.gov/offices/OSERS/OSEP/earlywrn.html.

50 Things You Can Do About Guns: A Citizen's Guide to Saving Lives and Stopping Gun Violence, James M. Murray (Robert D. Reed Publisher, 1994, $7.95). Information to help stop gun violence.

Gangs: The Epidemic Sweeping America, Fifth Edition. (Midwest Publishing, Inc., 21800 Haggerty Road, Suite 300, Northville MI 48167, 248-380-1700, 1994). Printed annually, usually distributed free-of-charge through local police and sheriff departments. This extensive review of gangs, their messages, activities, and dangers calls on professionals such as Carl S. Taylor, Ph.D., as well as police officers and other law enforcement officials nationwide, to prepare a frank and chilling picture of what schools and the broader community faces. Authorities say children first become involved with gangs at 13 years of age. Every school administrator should access this booklet.

Girls, Gangs, Women and Drugs, Carl S. Taylor (Michigan State University Press, 1993, $25.00). Through interviews and questionnaires, school girls and young women discuss their lives and interaction with the criminal justice system. Includes a slang glossary.

Keep Your Family Safe from Firearm Injury, American Academy of Pediatrics and Center to Prevent Handgun Violence (Free, send stamped, self-addressed legal-size envelope to STOP Brochure, 1225 Eye Street NW, Suite 1100, Washington, DC 20005, 202-289-7319). Brochure offers tips on how to reduce risks of firearm injury to families.

Kids and Gangs: What Parents and Educators Need to Know, Ann W. Lawson (Hazelden Information and Educational Services, 1994, $4.95). A complete picture of gangs: types of gangs, gang behavior, and psychological, social, and family dynamics factors that increase the risk of kids joining gangs. This is not a book for your teens.

National Coalition Against Domestic Violence, (PO Box 18749, Denver CO 80218, 303-839-1852, fax-303-831-9251). NCADV is dedicated to the empowerment of battered women and their children and to the elimination of personal and societal violence in the lives of women and their children. NCADV's work includes coalition building at the local, state, regional and national levels; public education and awareness activities; training and technical assistance; public policy development and monitoring; information and referral services. Provides links to direct state level and local services. Web site: www.ncadv.org.

National Crime Prevention Council, (Fulfillment Center, P.O. Box 1, 100 Church Street, Amsterdam, NY 12010, 800-NCPC-911). NCPC is a national non-profit organization whose mission is to help people prevent crime and build safer, stronger communities. The NCPC Web site, sponsored by Allstate Foundation and offered in English and Spanish, provides useful information about crime prevention, community building, comprehensive planning, and even fun stuff for kids. Visit McGruff the Crime Dog. Sections include: NCPC newsletter, local crime prevention initiatives, tips for neighborhood action, public service ads, teen safety, home safety, help for planning training events. Provides on-line ordering of books, videos, posters, and many free booklets/brochures. See *Stopping School Violence: 12 Things You Can Do* and *Safer Schools: Strategies for Educators and Law Enforcement*. Web site: www.ncpc.org.

National Domestic Violence Hotline: 800-799-SAFE, 800-787-3224-TDD. This Hotline answers about 10,000 calls each month from those experiencing domestic violence, as well as their family and friends. Provides callers with crisis intervention, information about domestic violence, and referrals to local programs 24 hours a day, 7 days a week in English and Spanish, with interpreters available to translate an additional 139 languages. The hotline offers: (1) *Crisis intervention* for helping the caller identify problems and possible solutions, including making plans for safety in an emergency;

(2) *Information about sources of assistance* for individuals and their friends, families, and employers wanting to learn more about domestic violence, child abuse, sexual assault, intervention programs for batterers, working through the criminal justice system, and related issues; and (3) *Referrals to battered women's shelters and programs*, social service agencies, legal programs, and other groups and organizations willing to help. The National Domestic Violence Hotline links individuals to help in their area using a nationwide database that includes detailed information on domestic violence shelters, other emergency shelters, legal advocacy and assistance programs, and social service programs.

National Runaway Switchboard: 800-621-4000, 800-621-0394-TDD. (3080 North Lincoln Avenue, Chicago IL 60657, 773-880-9860, fax-773-929-5150). A confidential hotline for runaway youth, teens in crisis, and concerned friends and family members. All services are free and available 24 hours every day. NRS services include: crisis intervention; message relay between runaways and their parent/legal guardian; referrals and conferences to community-based resources such as counseling, support groups, alternative housing, and health care; Home Free program in partnership with Greyhound Buslines, Inc. to help runaways return home to their families, and education and outreach services. E-mail address: info@nrscrisisline.org. Web site: www.nrscrisisline.org.

National Youth Gang Center, (Institute for Intergovernmental Research, P.O. Box 12739, Tallahassee, FL 32317, 800-446-0912, fax-850-386-5356). Assists state and local jurisdictions in the collection, analysis, and exchange of information on gang-related demographics, legislation, literature, research, and promising program strategies. Operated by U.S. Department of Justice. E-mail address: nygc@iir.com. Web Site: www.iir.com/nygc/.

Protecting the Gift: Keeping Children and Teenagers Safe, Gavin De Becker (The Dial Press/Random House, 1999, $22.95). De Becker is one of the country's leading experts on predicting violent behavior. In this indispensable resource, he provides keen insights into the behavior and strategies of predators. He offers practical new steps to enhance children's safety at every age level: specific questions parents can ask to screen effectively and evaluate baby-sitters, day-care services, schools, and doctors; a list of safety skills children need before being alone in public; warning signs to help parents protect children from sexual abuse; and how to keep teenage girls and boys from unsafe situations with peers and adults.

Safe at School: Awareness and Action for Parents, Carol Silverman Saunders (St. Martin's Press, 1999, $12.95). Each year in schools across the United States, more than 3 million crimes are committed, over 9,000 fires break out, and hundreds of thousands of students are injured. This book covers every school safety problem you can think of—guns, drugs, supervision, disaster preparation, sexual harassment, asbestos in the air, lead in the water, bullies, class trips, school maintenance, and many more. Step-by-step action plans explain how to identify safety problems at your child's school, how to form a parent safety group, and how to hold schools accountable for your child's safety.

Safeguarding Your Children, The National Parent-Teacher's Association (PTA) and The Allstate Foundation. (PTA: 330 N. Wabash Avenue, Suite 2100, Chicago, IL 60611-3690, 312-670-6782, 800-307-4PTA, fax-312-670-6783, 1995). Send publication inquiries to the attention of the customer service department. *Safeguarding Your Children* is a 30-page booklet full of information on how to help kids deal with all types of danger. Includes excellent resources. Available only through the PTA Web site. The Web site offers an extensive set of archives of pamphlets, publications, reports, handbooks, photographs, etc on a wide variety of subjects. Web site: www.pta.org (to get directly to the archives, go to www.pta.org/apta/archrs.htm.)

Teaching Tolerance Magazine, (Southern Poverty Law Center. 400 Washington Avenue, Montgomery AL 36104). Available to educators.

Traveler's Aid Society International: National Organization of Traveler's Aid Societies: 800-862-3723, (1612 K Street NW, Suite 506, Washington DC 20006, 202-546-1127, fax-202-546-9112). Serves individuals and families in crisis due to homelessness, mobility, or other disruptive circumstances. Web site: www.travelersaid.org.

"The Truths We Must Face to Curb Youth Violence," Amitai Etzioni, (*Education Week*, June 9, 1999). Amitai Etzioni is the University Professor at George Washington University. Professor Etzioni makes a compelling case for family involvement in character education. He also states his concerns about gun-loving lobbies, the role of the ACLU, TV violence, and how schools are working to prevent youth violence. He can be reached at etzioni@gwu.edu.

U.S. Department of Education 1998 Annual Report on School Safety. (U.S. Department of Education, ED Pubs, P.O. Box 1398, Jessup, MD 20794-1398, 877-4-ED-PUBS, 877-576-7734-TDD, fax-301-470-1244, Web site: www.ed.gov, on-line ordering available, free). Describes the nature and extent of crime and violence on school property. This report shows the measures that some schools have taken to prevent or address school violence and provides parents, students, and educators with information and resources to evaluate and enhance their own school's level of safety. It includes profiles of schools that have put in place programs and strategies that include school security, schoolwide education in violence prevention, counseling, and specialized student services. This is an outstanding resource. The full text of this publication can be found at www.ed.gov/pubs/AnnSchoolRept98.

Violence Against Women Office, (U.S. Department of Justice, Director Bonnie J. Campbell, 810 7th Street NW, Washington DC 20531, 202-616-8894, fax-202-307-3911, e-mail address: bcampbel@justice.usdoj.gov). Provides extensive information regarding violence against women, including: National Domestic Violence Hotline (see separate listing above), state domestic violence coalitions, newsletters, publications, press releases from the Executive Office of the U.S. Government, federal legislation, related research, grant programs, and related federal Web site resources. Web site: www.usdoj.gov/vawo.

Voices From The Streets: Young Former Gang Members Tell Their Stories, S. Beth Atkin (Little, Brown and Company, 1996, $17.95). This book presents the voices of young people who are rebuilding their lives after leaving a gang. They frankly reveal bits of their personal history, talk about their reasons for joining a gang, and recall what they experienced as a member—the good as well as the bad. They also explain why they quit and what it's like trying to stay out. Most speak of wishing parents had taken a more active role in their lives. Includes black and white photography.

When Men Batter Women: New Insights into Ending Abusive Relationships, Neil Jacobson and John Gottman (Simon & Schuster, 1998, $25.00). While national awareness of the issue of battering has increased in recent years, certain myths regarding abusive relationships still endure, including the idea that all batterers are alike. These two psychology professors and researchers offer a significant breakthrough in our understanding of the men who become batterers—and how to put a stop to the cycle of relationship violence.

CHAPTER 11
TEENS AND LIFE AFTER HIGH SCHOOL

Middle and high school students and their parents need to be involved in long term thinking regarding life plans following high school. This chapter highlights key factors in planning for a future, including information on technical, community, two-year and four-year colleges and vocational options. Much essential detailed information is provided in the text and in the extensive reference and resource section, including important foundational classes, tips for parental involvement in planning, timelines for college entrance exams, financial aid options, hot jobs for the 21st century, key questions to ask college admissions officers, advice on matching personalities with job types, and characteristics sought by employers.

CONNECT YOUR TEEN TO THE FUTURE

It is vital that parents and caregivers discuss career options and probe the important interests of the teen to help the teen understand how important it is to graduate from high school and to prepare for work, technical school, or college. You can discuss what your teen likes to do most, who he or she prefers to be with, which subjects are favorites, and where life can ideally go. Based on several serious discussions you and your adolescent will have, you can obtain ideas about the direction he or she needs to take and the information you both need to locate. You will want to help your teen try to connect realistically to specific education and job goals. Your talks will also provide incentives for sticking with high school.

See Your Teen's Counselor

High school and middle school counselors are busy professionals. It is important to stay informed about your son or daughter's academic programs. Monitor how the counselor and your adolescent are planning for a field of work, a college education, or a technical school in your teen's future. See the "Signposts" listing below to help give you an idea of the preparatory steps your teen should be taking. If college and technical education is planned, do not ignore this planning, or let it slip by. Insist on seeing the school counselor with your student if you have any questions. When you ask for time off to attend a scheduled conference with the school counselor advising your teen, impress upon your boss that you are dealing with your child's future. Indicate that your son or daughter may be among your company's future workers.

Signposts

FRESHMEN
- Plan tentative college-prep course schedule for next four years.
- Visit a local college and walk around to get a feel for the atmosphere.

SOPHOMORES
- Start browsing through your school's or local library's college guidebooks, attend a college fair, or explore the Internet.
- Send away for information from colleges you are interested in.
- October
  - Take the PSAT for practice.*

JUNIORS
- October
  - Take the PSAT.*
- Spring
  - Take the ACT or SAT I and SAT II subject tests.*
  - Make a preliminary short list of fewer than a dozen schools and visit as many as possible.
- Summer
  - Using your grade point average and test scores as guideposts, draw up your list of colleges and mail out requests for applications.

SENIORS
- Fall
  - Retake the ACT or SATs if not satisfied with your scores.*
  - Fill out your applications. Ask your English teacher or college counselor to proofread your essays. Give teachers plenty of time

to write letters of recommendation by asking them early in the
school year.
– Mail out completed applications.
– Wait.

* Standardized tests available to all high school students.
Reprinted with permission from *The Detroit Free Press*, Sunday, December 29, 1996. Reviewed for currency
1999 by Dr. Helene Mills, former Principal, Seaholm High School, Birmingham, Michigan.

Why College is Important

A two- or four-year college degree is becoming more and more important for un-
locking the doors to economic and educational opportunity in America today.
Getting a college education requires a lot of time, effort, and careful planning by
parents, students, and their counselors. It is well worth the effort, however, in that
it will provide knowledge and skills students will use for the rest of their lives to
help them succeed in whatever they undertake.

By Going to College Students:

- Get (and keep) a better job. Because the world is changing rapidly,
  and many jobs rely on new technology, more and more jobs require
  education beyond high school. With a two- or four-year college
  education, your child will have more jobs from which to choose.

- Earn more money. On average a person who goes to college earns
  more than a person who does not. Someone with a two-year
  associate degree earns more than a high school graduate. In 1996, a
  man with a college degree earned almost 96 percent more than a
  man with only a high school diploma, and a woman with a college
  degree earned almost 82 percent more than a woman with only a
  high school diploma.

- Get a good start to life. A college education helps your child acquire
  a wide range of knowledge in many subjects, as well as advanced
  knowledge in the specific subjects they are most interested in.
  Colleges train students to express thoughts clearly in speech and in
  writing, to make informed decisions, and to use technology-useful
  skills on and off the job.

Excerpted with permission from *Getting Ready for College Early*, Department
of Education, Partnership for Family Involvement in Education, 1999.

Students who are not interested in going to a four-year college or university for a bachelor's degree can benefit from the skills and knowledge that two years of college provide to compete in today's job market. These students may want to pursue a technical program in a community, junior, or technical college. These programs provide the skills and experience employers look for. Many high schools and some local employers offer career-focused programs called "Tech-prep." These programs coordinate high school course work with course work at local colleges, and in some cases give students the chance to learn in a real work setting.

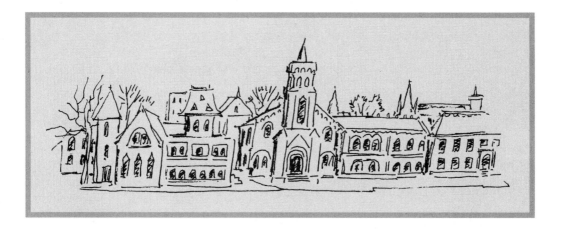

Taking the Right Courses Starts In Middle School

By the time your pre-teen is in sixth grade, families should start talking about going to college. Make it clear that you expect your children to go to college, and together start planning on how to get there. Everyone knows that high school courses and grades count for admission to college, but many people do not realize that a college education also builds on the knowledge and skills acquired in earlier years. Your child should plan a high school course schedule early, in the sixth or seventh grade.

Just as employers want workers who have certain skills, most colleges want students who have taken certain courses. Many of these courses can be taken only after a student has passed other, more basic courses. The most important thing a student can do to prepare for college is to sign up for the right middle and high school courses and work hard to pass them. College-bound middle and junior high school students should take:

- ALGEBRA I (in eighth grade) AND GEOMETRY (in ninth grade) or other challenging math courses that expect students to master the essentials of these subjects.
- ENGLISH, SCIENCE, AND HISTORY OR GEOGRAPHY. Together with math, these courses make up the "core" (the basic academic classes every student should take every year, in middle school and in high school).

- FOREIGN LANGUAGE. Many colleges require their students to study a foreign language for at least two years, and some prefer three or four years of one language.
- COMPUTER SCIENCE. Basic computer skills are now essential; more and more jobs require at least a basic knowledge of computers.
- THE ARTS. Many colleges view participation in the arts and music as a valuable experience that broadens students' understanding and appreciation of the world around them.

Excerpted with permission from *Getting Ready for College Early*, U.S. Department of Education, Partnership for Family Involvement in Education, 1999.

High School Courses Recommended for College

- ENGLISH— 4 years
  Types of classes: composition, American literature, English literature, world literature
- MATHEMATICS — 4 years
  Types of classes: algebra I, geometry, algebra II, trigonometry, precalculus, calculus
- HISTORY AND GEOGRAPHY — 2 to 3 years
  Types of classes: geography, U.S. history, U.S. government, world history, world culture, civics
- LABORATORY SCIENCE — 3 to 4 years
  Types of classes: biology, earth science, chemistry, physics
- VISUAL AND PERFORMING ARTS — 1 to 2 years
  Types of classes: art, dance, drama, music
- CHALLENGING ELECTIVES — 1 to 3 years
  Types of classes: economics, psychology, computer science, statistics, communications
- FOREIGN LANGUAGE — 3 to 4 years

Excerpted with permission from *Getting Ready for College Early*, U.S. Department of Education, Partnership for Family Involvement in Education, 1999.

SAVE ON TUITION

High school students can also take courses for credit at many colleges. These courses—Advanced Placement and Tech-prep—are available in the tenth, eleventh, and twelfth grades. Middle school and junior high school students who plan ahead and take algebra, a foreign language, and computer courses by the eighth grade are better prepared for Advanced Placement and Tech-Prep courses in high school.

More than 90 percent of today's high school seniors expect to attend college and more than 70 percent aspire to work in professional jobs, according to research conducted in the University of Chicago sociology department. But researchers

Barbara Schneider and David Stevenson, authors of a new book *The Ambitious Generation: America's Teenagers, Motivated but Directionless*, suggest these big dreams are not channeled into reality.

"Unfortunately, many adolescents make uninformed choices, and the cost of making them can be great," Schneider and Stevenson note. "Changing college majors several times, taking five years to complete a bachelor's degree, and finishing college not knowing what to do are some problems faced by young adults who make poor decisions based on too little information."

Preparation is of the essence because careers are changing at a rapid pace. Whole job classifications are eliminated by mergers, bankruptcies and globalization; technologies and market economies are shifting. Today's young people must find something they like. They must develop sound skills and flexible approaches toward pursuing their goals.

Too often, young people are still terrified by the "shoulds" told by their parents, teachers, friends, social class and other role models. This includes, "you should go to college," "you should earn a lot of money," "you should be a lawyer (a stockbroker, a nurse, an engineer) because your parent or grandparent worked in that field."

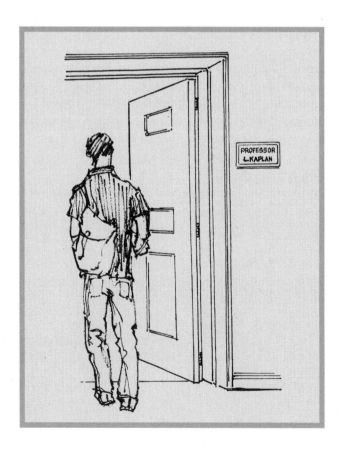

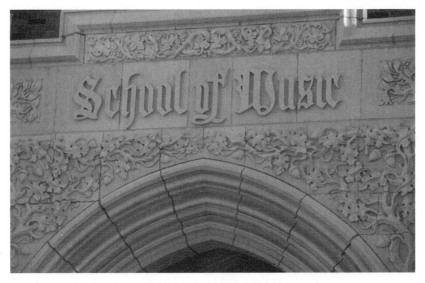

Parents need to provide encouragement to adolescents who choose a different field of study than that of other family members. Independent thinking is an important learning task.

IDENTIFY TYPES OF PEOPLE AND SKILLS

Louise Welsh Schrank, author of *How to Choose the Right Career,* suggests that teens are better prepared for career decisions by identifying their favorite types of people and skills. She suggests the following indicators:

- BODY WORKERS: Often including athletes, physical education instructors, and "blue collar" workers, these people work with tools or machines in skilled trades, outdoor, technical or service jobs. Body workers are typically practical, rugged, athletic, healthy and aggressive.
- DATA DETAIL: Part of the "white collar" or office workers, these people hold jobs involving clerical or numerical tasks, such as banking, bookkeeping, data processing, and accounting. These workers are usually good at following instructions and attending carefully to detail work.
- PERSUADERS: Usually holding management or sales positions, these workers have jobs where they persuade people to perform some kind of action, such as buying goods and services.
- SERVICE WORKERS: Frequently working in education, health care, or social welfare, these workers hold jobs where they teach, heal, or help people. Hairdressers, waiters, instructors, health care workers, and tour guides are part of this group.
- CREATIVE ARTISTS: These people work with words, music, or art in a creative way. Actors, musicians, composers, authors, and sculptors are in this group.

- INVESTIGATORS: Usually performing scientific or laboratory work, investigators research how the world is put together and how to solve problems.

Reprinted from *How to Choose the Right Career* by Louise Welsh Schrank. Used with permission of NTC/Contemporary Publishing Group, Inc.

LEARNING ABOUT A CAREER

Once your teen has identified an interesting career area, take time to help your adolescent learn more about what jobs in this field are really like. Marty Nemko, author of *Cool Careers For Dummies®*, suggests looking at the U.S. Department of Labor/Bureau of Statistic's *Occupational Outlook Handbook*, which not only lists careers but also describes whether the demand for employees is increasing or decreasing. With the help of a researcher at a local public library, teens can check with the U.S. Bureau of Labor Statistics and the Higher Education Research for career descriptions. Students can locate information about starting salaries and the fastest growing careers.

Once your teen identifies an interest in a specific field of work, you and your teen need to find out what education is needed. Students can interview people who are doing jobs in the field by contacting professional associations and asking for referrals. These associations are glad to share their experience with young people. Many people will allow your teen to "shadow" them for a day. Do not be shy; ask among friends and professionals whom you know, along with anyone who works in your teen's area of interest. Guidance counselors can suggest mentors in the field of choice for your adolescent. Your son or daughter can always check an association's Web site, and check bookstores to review titles and topics about their chosen field.

Hot Jobs of the 21st Century	Annual Salary		
Chief Information Officer	$100,000	–	$200,000
Wireless Engineer	80,000	–	120,000
Software-Development Manager	60,000	–	100,000
Database Manager	60,000	–	80,000
Director of E-commerce	50,000	–	80,000
Webmaster	50,000	–	70,000
Tool-and-Die Worker	40,000	–	70,000
Teacher Trainer	35,000	–	60,000
Telemarketer/Customer Rep.	20,000	–	35,000

Reprinted from "*Your Next Job*" from *Newsweek*, February 1, 1999.
Used with permission of *Newsweek*.

Fastest-growing jobs, 1996 - 2006	Percentage increase
Database Manager	118%
Computer Engineer	109
Systems Analyst	103
Personal/Home Aide	85
Physical Therapy Assistant	79
Home Health Aide	76
Medical Assistant	74
Desktop Publisher	74
Physical Therapist	71
Occupational Therapist	69

Reprinted from "*Your Next Job*" from *Newsweek*, February 1, 1999. Used with permission of *Newsweek*.

Get Experience

With the price of clothes, cars, and college spiraling upwards, many young people seek part-time employment. The most common jobs are fast-food server, retail clerk, or lawn maintenance worker. Nearly any job can provide a learning experience. It is important that your adolescent restrict their hours to provide adequate study time, rest, and develop good saving habits to seed their college account.

The National Longitudinal Study of Adolescent Health (Add Health Study), found that students who worked 20 hours or more per week were more likely to experience emotional distress and to use harmful substances.

Stephen Hamilton, professor at Cornell University, says that parents should be as concerned about where their teenagers work as they are about their schools. He indicates that youth employment can have either profoundly positive or seriously harmful effects on adolescents. In a recent report for the National Resource Council and the Institute of Medicine, Hamilton and his colleagues are calling for criteria for school related and publicly supported job programs.

"Years of research at Cornell University has shown that good-quality youth apprenticeships, internships, and jobs can improve students' career paths by teaching personal, social, and technical competencies in the workplace as well as self-esteem," says Hamilton.

Both school personnel and parents must monitor work places for safety, hours of employment, and learning possibilities. Otherwise time should be spent preparing for the future with study, volunteering, and youth activities.

"Retail jobs can provide an advanced degree in experience," said a marketing consultant recently. "They can provide the kind that will help ratchet young people above others who are working for glamorous companies doing work that does not challenge their brains. Small stores are learning laboratories where young people can experience a whole vista of retailing: handling customers, overseeing stock levels, handling returns, and mailings."

Still more high school and college students are investing time to help the less fortunate. Break Away, an eight-year-old organization based in Nashville, estimates 20,000 students in spring of 1999 will have crisscrossed North America to help the poor and the sick. According to *U.S. News and World Report*, the charitable venture not only helps to clean homeless shelters and distribute food, it provides real world experience to impress colleges and future employers. The experience also promotes social responsibility in your teen.

> Both school personnel and parents must monitor work places for safety, hours of employment, and learning possibilities.

Your adolescent may find career insight through participation in student activities, such as debate, student council, vocational clubs, theater or music. Such activities also provide positive mentoring by adults.

Do not discount what a teen reads or what Web sites he or she visits regularly, as contributing to a positive future. Billionaire computer giant Bill Gates started his career by fixing computers and movie mogul Stephen Spielberg produced short films in high school.

In their book, *The 500 Year Delta*, futurists Jim Taylor and Watts Wacker write: "We look at the World Wide Web . . . and we see . . . a global 'freedom to know' – a world in which for the first time in human history, caste or schooling or economic circumstance no longer limits access to knowledge, a world in which knowledge itself is less important than the skill to access it." Be sure your adolescent is skillful in using the Internet.

EDUCATION FOR THE CAREER CHOSEN

The next challenge is deciding where to go for additional education. Researchers Schneider and Stevenson warn of "ambition paradox" which occurs when students with high ambitions choose an educational route with low odds of success.

For example, a teen with technical interests might be better served at a trade school where he or she could cultivate an ability to work with his hands, solve technical problems and interfacing with customers. Over 1,000 vocational/trade schools offer two- and four-year technical degrees in such diverse fields as professional tennis management, performance engine mechanics and refrigeration, heating and ventilation.

For teens who have an interest in information technologies (IT)—the world of computers—there are an ever increasing number of educational and vocational possibilities. Many technical support programs, teaching skills for basic personal computer or network system support, are only six months to one year in length. Many computer-programming languages can be learned in six months or less.

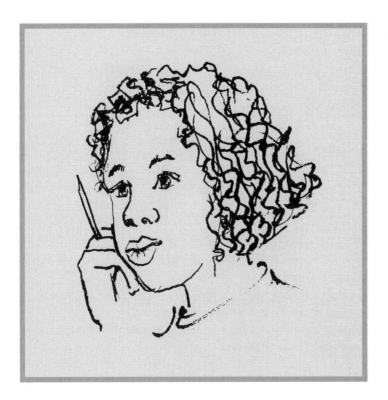

Often, computer and software development companies offer paid training programs for these skills to interested students. Many IT educational programs offer paid work internships in real job settings, where basic skills can be greatly expanded. New technologies emerge monthly, creating new jobs, such as Web site design, e-commerce, and virtual reality research and development. There is a constant and growing shortage of skilled workers to fill IT jobs, which makes it easy for students to move easily from training programs to good paying jobs.

If your teen chooses a college path, select several options among the 3,500 colleges and universities in America. Keep in mind your adolescent is competing against 2.6 million graduating seniors. The best schools have an abundant pool of qualified applicants.

"The top colleges shape a pool of incoming freshmen," said one director of college counseling. "They seek a balance between men and women, a geographic balance, a diversity culturally and ethnically. They may seek special talents for programming on their campuses. Keep in mind this criteria could shift from year to year." High school guidance counselors, guidebooks, and Web sites will be a big help (see the REFERENCES AND RESOURCES section at the end of this chapter). Remember you are busy, and your teen is very busy, but watch for college admission filing dates and help your teen keep the process on track. Following are important questions for your adolescent to think out before going to college interviews.

Questions For College Admissions Officers

- When must I choose a major?
- What types of internships/co-op experiences are available?
- How can I arrange a campus visit? Are there any special visitation days on your campus coming up?
- What are the application deadlines for admission and financial aid?
- How tough will it be to earn a degree in four years? What percentage of a typical freshman class will actually graduate from your college?
- How many freshmen courses are taught by graduate students instead of full-fledged professors? What is the typical class size?
- What weighs most heavily in deciding whether a student gets accepted or not?
- What is the average high school grade point average (GPA) of the entering freshmen class, and what is their average GPA after freshman year?
- How do you assign faculty advisors to students, especially those who are undecided about their majors?
- What academic services do you offer to students (tutoring, career counseling, study skills workshops)?

From *College Planning For Dummies*® by Pat Ordovensky. Copyright© 1997 IDG Books Worldwide, Inc. All rights reserved. Reproduced here by permission of the publisher. *For Dummies* is a registered trademark of IDG Books Worldwide, Inc.

How Colleges Evaluate Candidates

Every college uses a scoring system to rank its applicants, according to Pat Ordovensky, author of *College Planning For Dummies*®. This Scoring System is as follows:

- Unweighted grade point average (unweighted means all your student's course marks averaged together)
- Honors, advanced placement courses
- SAT and ACT test scores
- Extracurricular activities
- Teacher and counselor recommendations
- Content and writing style of student's essay

From *College Planning For Dummies*® by Pat Ordovensky. Copyright© 1997 IDG Books Worldwide, Inc. All rights reserved. Reproduced here by permission of the publisher. *For Dummies* is a registered trademark of IDG Books Worldwide, Inc.

Some colleges also give points for class rank and impressions formed during an interview. Then each item gets a score, say on a scale of one to six, and the sub-scores are added for a total. At other colleges, if your first score is high enough, you're an automatic "admit." If it's too low, you're a "deny." It's not unusual for an admissions committee to consider candidates in descending order of their scores and stop when they have enough candidates.

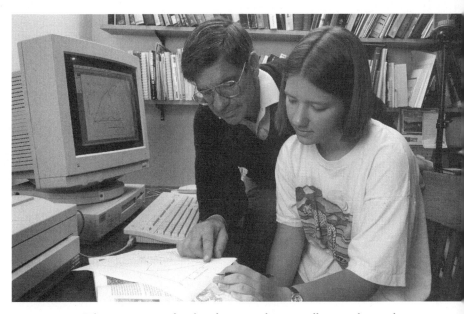

When your son or daughter begins applying to colleges, make sure he or she also completes the Free Application for Federal Student Aid (FAFSA) and other financial aid forms required. The FAFSA may be completed on-line at http://www.FAFSA.ed.gov.

SEARCHING FOR FINANCIAL AID

You and your teen need to start now to search out financial aid options to augment your savings. Numerous educators confirm that wherever there is a will there is a way to get into school. Financial aid is plentiful, along with tuition grants, work-study programs and other enhancements.

When your son or daughter begins applying to colleges, make sure he or she also completes the Free Application for Federal Student Aid (FAFSA) and other financial aid forms required by the college. These forms must be completed well in advance of the financial aid deadlines. Missing a deadline by only one day can cost your family thousands of dollars in scholarships and other forms of financial aid.

It is wise to file the FAFSA even though you have not completed your final income tax return. Estimated income figures may be used and corrected later. Families who wait beyond the deadline will likely have missed many financial aid opportunities. The FAFSA may be competed on-line at http://www.FAFSA.ed.gov (see REFERENCES AND RESOURCES section at end of chapter).

Some families choose not to file the form each year their student is in college. This is a mistake. Income is only one of the factors used to determine a student's financial aid eligibility. For example, the number of family members attending college, business losses, and high family medical expenses are all taken into account in determining eligibility.

In addition to applying for federal, state, and college-sponsored scholarships and grants, your son or daughter can check with the service clubs in your community for the possibility of obtaining a scholarship application. Among many opportunities, three national groups that offer scholarships to women are the American Association of University Women (AAUW), the American Business Women's Association (ABWA), and Soroptimists International. You may also want to check with your local Lions Club, Kiwanis Club, or Rotary Club. Criteria for these awards vary.

Private scholarships are available from a variety of sources (these are listed in several books and on Web sites—see REFERENCES AND RESOURCES). Beware of scholarship services that guarantee a scholarship for a hefty fee. Scholarship scams have become increasingly prevalent in recent years, and the Federal Trade Commission (FTC) has become very aggressive in prosecuting offenders. The National Fraud Information Center may be contacted at 1-800-876-7060.

Federal Financial Aid

Federal financial aid programs provide nearly 70 percent of financial aid funds, colleges and universities provide 20 percent, and state and private sources provide 10 percent. Seek out information on financial aid sources early in the financial aid process to obtain a basic understanding of the programs and eligibility criteria.

Almost all federal aid is driven by the FAFSA. This form will tell you whether your teen qualifies for a subsidized or unsubsidized loan. As a general rule of thumb, students do not have to pay back grants or scholarships. Students do have to pay back loans. Several federal programs are described below.

- STAFFORD LOANS: These are federal loans that come in subsidized and unsubsidized versions. The government picks up the interest on subsidized Stafford loans while the student is enrolled at least half-time in school. On unsubsidized loans, the interest accumulates while the student is in school, though the payments can be deferred until the student is out of school. While subsidized loans go to needy students, those who have no need can get an unsubsidized Stafford loan. Interest rates are capped at 8.25 percent.
- PERKINS LOANS: Designed for high-need students, these subsidized loans make up the best loan package available for students. Interest is capped at 5 percent.
- PELL GRANTS: These outright gifts are designed for students with high need. There are no academic criteria for these grants. The student must demonstrate need and be enrolled in an eligible institution. The maximum grant for 1999-2000 is $3,125.
- SUPPLEMENTAL EDUCATIONAL OPPORTUNITY GRANTS (SEOG's): These grants do not have to be paid back, are targeted at high-need students, and are not based on merit.

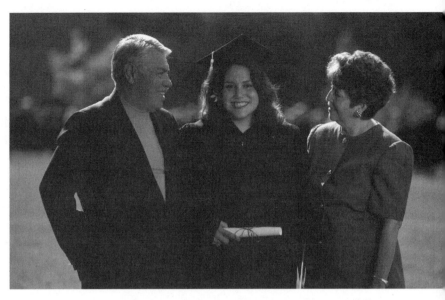

It is hard to replace the joy that occurs when your student successfully completes study to abtain a college education. Encourage and plan with your son or daughter to enroll in advanced study after high school.

- FEDERAL WORK-STUDY PROGRAM: Colleges are awarded funds that the student can earn by working in such areas as food service, the library, the computer center, or offices. These programs are based on need. The student earns the amount of the aid by working while attending school, and this money does not have to be paid back after graduation.

- AMERICORPS: A federal community service program in which volunteers receive living allowances and contributions for college costs for 1,700 hours of annual service. For information, call 800-942-2677.

- PLUS LOAN: Most families are eligible for the federal PLUS Loan which provides financial assistance to make up the difference between the student's cost of education and the financial aid received. The interest rate is variable, with a cap of 9 percent and a minimum monthly repayment of $50. Detailed information on the PLUS Loan may be obtained by writing to or calling the Federal Student Aid Information Center (see REFERENCES AND RESOURCES section at end of chapter).

WORK IS CHANGING; CHARACTERISTICS NEEDED

Some children know what they want to do for a living by the time they finish middle school, such as a 12-year-old Webmaster or 14-year-old caterer for teen parties. But most young people are not that lucky.

Parents often tend to nudge their children toward a career path they wish they could have pursued—doctor, lawyer, or statistician—or expect school counselors to channel them in the right direction. Adults assume that getting their children into the right college will provide answers, or connections that will lead to life skills and lucrative offers. College students may wind up falling into careers more by chance than by choice. There has to be a better way.

Today's careers are changing more rapidly than channels on a cable-equipped television set. "The fastest growing occupations between now and 2006 are projected to be database administrators, computer support specialists, and all other computer scientists, followed by computer engineers, systems analysts, and personal and home health care aides," according to the Bureau of Labor Statistics' *1998-1999 Occupational Outlook Handbook*.

The most striking—and challenging—feature of the new world of work is how much it will demand of young people in terms of study, flexibility, and long hours. Consider that 8 million people held down more than one job in 1997, compared with 3.8 million multiple jobholders in 1970.

Just a decade ago, expertise in a single discipline, like engineering, was enough to develop a comfortable future at a corporation. Today the best candidates have a grounding in several languages, keen computer and communications skills, and an ability to adapt to frequent shake-ups, mergers, and bankruptcies in the business world.

This chapter and the REFERENCES AND RESOURCES section following the chapter will help parents and caregivers more easily take up the task of helping their adolescent prepare for work after high school. As U.S. Secretary of Education Richard W. Riley says: "We have a responsibility to our children. While they represent only 20 percent of our population, children are 100 percent of America's future. They are our greatest investment, and it's up to us to help them understand the importance of investing in themselves."

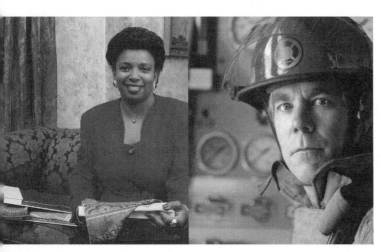

There are a wide range of opportunities for work that is valuable, enjoyable, and demanding. Advanced training and education will be needed for nearly every job in the 21st century.

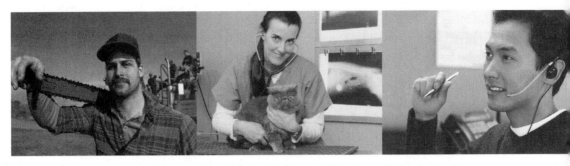

In this country, opportunities abound for work that is challenging and stimulating. Be sure your teen knows about the many choices available and prepares well to reach his or her chosen goal.

Eyes on the Prize

In making decisions about work, technical school, or college, keep in mind that the outcome is to enrich your teen's mind and strengthen possibilities for employment. These are characteristics that employers seek:

- PROBLEM SOLVERS: people who look for every option to solve a problem and do not go around complaining or blaming others.
- SIFTERS AND SORTERS: people who use their brains to make sense of the puzzles in the workplace, who know how to research and apply what they learn.
- HEADS THAT FOCUS ON THE BOTTOM-LINE: workers who are out for results.
- PEOPLE WHO SPEAK AND WRITE WELL: workers who can get their point across clearly using the best choice of words, correct grammar, and spelling.
- TEAM PLAYERS WHO CAN LISTEN: people who work well with others, and want to help everyone win.
- PEOPLE WHO WELCOME NEW TECHNOLOGIES: workers who can figure out ways to use new technologies to reach the company's goals.
- IDEA PEOPLE WHO ARE CREATIVE: people who try new ways of getting the job done.
- LEADERS WHO HAVE INSIGHT INTO WHAT THE FUTURE MAY BRING: people with self-confidence and pride in themselves and their own judgement.
- SURFERS ON THE THIRD WAVE: learners who understand how fast change occurs and can handle it well.
- ORGANIZERS AND DEVELOPERS: people who can motivate and manage others and are good at directing and producing the best products and services.

What are Employers Looking for When They Hire? adapted with permission from *Where Do I Fit In?* from The Pryor Report Management Newsletter, October, 1994 (P.O. Box 101, Clemson, SC 29633, 800-237-7967).

REFERENCES AND RESOURCES

College Guides

America's Best Colleges: The 1999 Directory of Colleges and Universities, Mortimer B. Zuckerman, ed. (U.S. News Specialty Marketing, 1998, $5.95).

An Insider's Guide to Success in the Two-Year College, Gary Sattelmeyer (Barron's Educational Series, 1999, $8.95). This guide has been written by someone who regularly meets, greets, and advises students in two-year colleges—someone who is on the inside. Includes an appendix that lists all of the accredited two-year colleges in the U.S.

Barron's Best Buys in College Education, 5th Edition, Lucia Solorzano (Barron's Educational Series, 1998, $14.95). This practical and useful book profiles nearly 300 private and public U.S. college bargains. The author points out that it is not true that quality always comes with a high price tag among universities. The guide has "quick lists" to help the reader target what they are looking for related to university size, focus, atmosphere, and tuition rate. There follows a set of alphabetical in-depth profiles of universities, including information on student/faculty ratio, faculty qualifications, financial aid availability, student demographics, and more.

Barron's Compact Guide to Colleges, 11th Edition, (Barron's Educational Series, 1998, $8.95). This shorter and smaller college directory lists and describes approximately 400 major schools across the United States. All profiles have been taken from the new 23rd edition of *Barron's Profiles of American Colleges*.

Barron's Profiles of American Colleges, 23rd Edition, (Barron's Educational Series, 1998, $25.00, book and disk). Updated for the 1998-99 school year, the newest edition of the nation's definitive college directory presents profiles of every accredited four-year college in all 50 states. Two disks (one for Windows and one for the Mac) give abridged profiles of each school listed in the book.

Barron's Profiles of American Colleges on CD-ROM (Barron's Educational Series, 1998, $34.95).

Fiske Guide to Colleges 1999, Edward B. Fiske (Times Books, 1998, $20.00). Fiske is a former education editor for the *New York Times*. Rather than trying to offer a comprehensive guide to the nation's colleges, the *Fiske Guide to Colleges 1999* focuses on the "best and most interesting colleges and universities" and offers in-depth profiles supported by clearly presented statistics. Each of the more than 300 schools selected is rated in terms of three major themes: academics, social life, and quality of life.

Four-Year Colleges 2000 (Peterson's, 1999, $26.95). This highly respected source of information features fact-filled profiles of more than 2,000 colleges and universities and college-search indices on CD for quick state-by-state comparisons.

The Insider's Guide to Colleges 1999, 25th Edition, Staff of *Yale Daily News*, (St. Martin's Griffin, 1998, $16.99). Written by students for students, this guide gives candid, in-depth profiles of more than 300 schools in all 50 states and Canada, with emphasis on academic strengths and weaknesses, faculty, housing and food, social life, extracurricular activities, and more.

A National Directory of Four-Year Colleges, Two-Year Colleges, and Post-High School Training Programs for Young People with Learning Disabilities, P.M. Fielding (Partners in Publishing, 1994, $29.95).

Peterson's Competitive Colleges, 1999-2000, 18th Edition, (Peterson's Guides, 1999, $18.95). Cited as "the most accurate guide to undergraduate institutions" by a survey of college administrators, this fact-filled annual presents in-depth profiles of more than 350 U.S. colleges and universities that attract and admit the world's best students.

College Financial Aid

College Student's Guide to Merit and Other No-Need Funding: 1998-2000 (Reference Service Press). Scholarships are available even to students who do not come from lower-income families. Corporate sponsorships are awarded by businesses, industry groups and unions to children—and sometimes other relatives—of company employees. Some schools offer merit or Presidential scholarships to top students, regardless of need.

Don't Miss Out: The Ambitious Student's Guide to Financial Aid 1998-1999, Anna Leider and Robert Leider (Octameron Associates, 1998, $8.00). For more than 20 years, *Don't Miss Out* has been a widely used, authoritative book on financing a college education. Written from a consumer's point of view, this new edition presents everything students and their parents should know, listing hundreds of scholarship, grant and loan sources. Charts, tables, and easy worksheets guide students and parents through the financial maze.

FASTweb.com: A Web site which provides a free, searchable database of more than 400,000 private sector scholarships, grants, and loans. Web site: www.fastweb.com.

Federal Student Financial Aid Information Center, 800-801-0576. Provides the most up-to-date information about student aid supplied by the U.S. Department of Education. You can also get a copy of the federal financial aid form, which is required to apply for all federal financial aid, or complete the free application on-line at http://fafsa.ed.gov.

Financial Aid Financer: Expert Answers to College Financing Questions, 10th Edition, Joseph M. Re (Octameron Associates, 1998, $6.00).

FinAid: The Smart Student Guide to Financial Aid. This Web site offers extensive information on student loans, financial aid resources, financial aid application forms, scholarship service scam alerts, and much more. FinAid was created by Mark Kantrowitz, a noted financial aid and college planning author. Web site: www.finaid.org.

The Financial Aid Book: The Insider's Guide to Private Scholarships, Grants, and Fellowships, 3rd Edition, Student Financial Services, ed. (Perpetual Press, 1999, $24.95). This book provides information for over 3,000 private scholarships, grants, and fellowships. Students will be able to follow each step in the application process from requesting information to filling out financial aid forms and writing winning essays.

The Government Financial Aid Book: The Insider's Guide to State and Federal Government Grants and Loans (Serial), Student Financial Services, ed. (Perpetual Press, 1999, $14.95). This book simplifies the confusing application process by helping the reader understand each program and by providing detailed instructions and tips for completing forms. Samples of actual forms are included and a unique award index helps students find scholarships that best apply to their situation.

Kaplan Financial Aid Web Site, Provides much information regarding student loans, financial planning for college, admissions timelines, on-line ordering of books and software. Web site: www.kaploan.com.

National Association for College Admission Counseling Fair, 703-836-2222, Web site: www.nacac.com. For western U.S. fairs, contact the Rocky Mountain Association for College Admission Counseling Fairs, 505-835-5424.

The Prentice Hall Guide to Scholarships and Fellowships for Math and Science Students: A Resource for Students Pursuing Careers in Mathematics and Science, Mark Kantrowitz (Prentice Hall Trade, 1993, $29.95).

Project EASI: Easy Access for Students and Institutions. Government, education, student and business leaders initiated this Web site as a collaborative effort to use cutting-edge technology and business processes to dramatically transform the administration of student financial aid and improve customer access to information and funding for education beyond high school. Provides much information on federal aid programs. Students can file their Free Application for Federal Student Aid (FAFSA) on-line at this site. Web site: http://easi.ed.gov.

The Student Guide 1999-2000 (U.S. Department of Education, 800-433-3243, Federal Student Aid Information Center, P.O. Box 84, Washington, DC 20044-0084, 800-4FED-AID). Free. Provides an extensive and annually updated discussion of all federal student aid programs. Web site: www.ed.gov/prog_info/SFA/Student Guide.

School and Work Success

The Ambitious Generation: America's Teenagers, Motivated but Directionless, Barbara Schneider and David Stevenson. (Yale University Press, 1999, $26.00). The authors, both sociologists, reveal that modern teenagers are not only misdirected, but often very alienated. Shows how parents and teachers can take adolescents' admirable raw ambition and provide them with direction and social support.

Barron's How to Prepare for the ACT: American College Testing Program Assessment, George Ehrenshaft, Robert L. Lehrman, Fred Obrecht, and Allan Mundsack (Barron's Educational Series, 1998, $14.95). Revised and updated to reflect the most recent ACT college entrance tests, this manual presents a full-length diagnostic test and four complete model exams, all with questions answered and explained.

Barron's SAT I: How to Prepare for SAT I, Samuel Brownstein, Mitchel Weiner, and Sharon Weiner Green (Barron's Educational Series, 20th Ed., 1998, $13.95). Extensively revised and updated, this new edition of this best-selling test prep manual presents one complete diagnostic test and seven full-length model SAT I tests, with answer keys, explanations, and solutions. New to this edition are explanations of dozens of essential test-taking tactics.

Break Away®, (Box 6026, Station B, Nashville TN 37235, 615-343-0385, fax-615-343-3255.) *Break Away's®* mission is to promote service on the local, regional, national and international levels through college break-oriented programs which immerse students in often vastly different cultures, to heighten social awareness and advocate life-long social action. E-mail Address: breakaway@ alternativebreaks.com. Web site: www.alternativebreaks.com.

Careers in the Food Services Industry, Robert Otterbourg (Barron's Educational Series, 1999, $9.95). This book provides an analysis of the trends in the culinary world, with insight into the types of school and training programs available for someone interested in working in some segment of the industry. Culinary occupations are profiled, including chef, baker, caterer, restauranteur, and employee of a chain restaurant or institutional kitchen.

Careers in Healthcare, Robert Wilson (Barron's Educational Series, 1999, $9.95). The healthcare field is filled with opportunities for those people who have an interest but not a degree, for jobs such as dental assistant, emergency medical technician, licensed practical nurse, and physical therapy aide. This book details the variety of employment opportunities in the healthcare industry, how to determine career paths that are a good fit, and where to go to get the right training.

Clicking: 17 Trends That Drive Your Business—And Your Life, Faith Popcorn and Lys Marigold (Harperbusiness, 1998, $14.00). Nobody has been more accurate in demonstrating how to profit from tracking the trends, and in *Clicking*, Popcorn describes how to click into more recently identified trends to future-fit oneself professionally and personally. *Clicking* is an invaluable road map to the newest lifestyle trends.

College Planning For Dummies®, by Pat Ordovensky. (IDG Books Worldwide, 1999, $19.99). The process of selecting a college, applying for admission and dealing with finances can be an overwhelming and frustrating experience for students and parents alike. With more than 3,500 colleges and universities in the U.S. to choose from, this book guides the reader through the planning, research, and selection process. For more information about this and other titles published by IDG Books Worldwide, call 800-762-2974 or visit their Web sites at www.dummies.com and www.idgbooks.com.

Cool Careers For Dummies®, Marty Nemko and Paul and Sarah Edwards. (IDG Books Worldwide, 1998, $16.99). The cool careers yellow pages features 500-plus career profiles of emerging and fun occupations, along with answering the 20 most revealing questions to help identify the best career for your adolescent or yourself.

Family Life and School Achievement: Why Poor Black Children Succeed or Fail, Reginald M. Clark (University of Chicago Press, 1984, $9.95). Compares the backgrounds of high achieving inner city teenagers with peers who are failing, and determines what makes the difference.

Finding Your Perfect Work: The New Career Guide to Making a Living, Creating a Life, Paul and Sarah Edward (JP Tarcher, 1996, $16.95). A *What Color Is Your Parachute?* for the next decade, *Finding Your Perfect Work* helps readers define what they really want in life and lists over 1,600 self-employment occupations with rating scales for determining their suitability to readers' personal styles, resources, and lifestyle needs.

"For '99 College Applicant, Stiffest Competition Ever," Ethan Bronner. *New York Times*, July 12, 1999. The 1999 college application season was the most competitive in U.S. history, with indications that the trend

will intensify in the next 10 years. Check the *New York Times* on-line at www.nytimes.com or visit your local library. Important reading.

Getting Ready for College Early: A Handbook for Parents of Students in Middle and Junior High School Years, U.S. Department of Education and Partnership for Family Involvement in Education. See U.S. Department of Education listing below for contact information. This guidebook will help you and your children understand the steps you need to take during the middle and junior high school years to get ready for college.

The Gifted Kids Survival Guide: A Teen Handbook, Judy Galbraith and Jim Delisle (Free Spirit Publishing, 1996, $14.95). Facts, findings, and insights about giftedness, intelligence testing, and IQ; school survival, success, and learning; goal-setting, planning for the future, and college preparation.

How to Choose the Right Career, by Louise Welsh Schrank (VGM Career Horizons. 1991, $11.95) This field-tested workbook helps career enthusiasts examine today's and tomorrow's job markets, identify skills, and compare and evaluate the education and training available.

Imagine the Future: A Teenager's Guide to the Next Century and Beyond and *Parent's Guide—Imagine the Future: Helping Your Teen Prepare for the Future*, Joseph Malgeri (Career Solutions, 1997, $8.95). The world is changing too fast for most to realize the implications on teens who will leave school between 2000 and 2005 to enter the work force. These two resources give teens and parents a clear picture of what work will be like, the skills teens will need and whose responsibility it is to prepare.

Learning a Living: A Guide to Planning Your Career and Finding a Job for People with Learning Disabilities, Attention Deficit Disorder, and Dyslexia, Dale S. Brown (Woodbine House, 1999, $18.95). Written by an author who grew up with learning disabilities, this book discusses finding a job that emphasizes strengths and minimizes the effects of a learning disability. It addresses career issues for high schoolers, college students, and adults with learning disabilities, dyslexia, and attention deficit disorder.

Life's A Trip: Get Packed and Prepared for the 21st Century, Jill Davis. (1078 Covington Road, Bloomfield MI 48301, 248-642-7582, $30.00) A vocational counselor prepares a workbook to help students explore values, abilities, interests, and aptitudes. Information on the college application process and technical training. Parents/caregivers, schools and students will find this workbook invaluable. Two hundred packed pages.

Occupational Outlook Handbook, U.S. Department of Labor/Bureau of Statistics. (VGM Career Books, 1996, $22.95). A comprehensive, respected career reference offers up-to-date information on two hundred different occupations for job seekers looking for quick information on employment opportunities, qualifications, salaries, working conditions, and career advances.

Preparing Students for the 21st Century, Donna Uchida, Marvin Cetron and Floretta McKenzie (American Association of School Administrators Distribution Center, 1996, $15.95). What families and schools can do to help prepare teens for success in the 21st century.

"Preparing Your Child for College", Consumer Information Center, Preparing Your Child for College, Pueblo, CO 81009. Free handbook.

Student Success Secrets, Eric Jensen and Tom Kerr (illustrator) (Barron's Educational Series, 1996, $8.95). Sure-fire study strategies that can increase test scores and raise grades dramatically. Advice on developing motivation to learn. Good-humored and approachable style with cartoons included.

Teaching the New Basic Skills: Principles for Educating Children to Thrive in a Changing Economy, Richard J. Murane and Frank Levy (Free Press, 1996, $24.00). Drawing on the work of real teachers, parents, and administrators, this book provides a blueprint for turning our schools around.

Think College Early Web site. Linked to the main U.S. Department of Education Web site, this site provides information and publications for students, parents, educators, and the community to help them to think about and plan for college in the middle school years. Web site: www.ed.gov/think college/early.

U.S. Department of Education, (400 Maryland Avenue SW, Washington DC 20202, 800-USA-LEARN, 800-437-0833-TTY, fax-202-401-0689, 877-4ED-PUBS, toll free for publications). E-mail Address: CustomerService@inet.ed.gov. Web site: www.ed.gov.

What Smart Students Know: Maximum Grades, Optimum Learning, Minimum Time, Adam Robinson (Crown
Publishers Inc., 1993, $16.00). Starting from the premise that successful students are not necess-
arily any more brilliant than their less successful peers, but have simply mastered the art of
efficient learning, Adam Robinson introduces high school and college students to an innovative
approach that can help them achieve top grades while discovering the joy of true learning.
Contains hundreds of practical tips about "maximum grades, optimum learning, minimum time."

"Your Next Job," *Newsweek*, February 1, 1999. Excellent article that explores how careers are changing
as we move into the 21st century.

The Winner-Take-All Society: Why the Few at the Top Get So Much More Than the Rest of Us, Robert H. Frank
and Philip J. Cook (Penguin USA, 1996, $13.95). An analysis of "Winner-Take-All" markets and the
jobs that are created and won by the elite.

CHAPTER 12
TEENS AND A BETTER COMMUNITY

Good news! Both adults and the young people who read *Healthy Teens* can be encouraged by the continued research that shows that, even if faced with almost impossible odds in early life, individuals can grow up and be successful. The research comes from life-span development studies in the sixties and earlier, that followed children born into seriously difficult conditions such as in families where parents were mentally ill, alcoholic, abusive, criminal, or in communities that were poverty-stricken or war torn. The early findings from these long term studies is that at least 50 percent, and often 70 percent, of young people in these conditions overcome odds and grow up to lead successful lives. This chapter discusses resiliency in adolescents and programs that assist in building strength—another term for resiliency—in teens.

RESILIENCY DEFINED

Bonnie Benard, a researcher in the resiliency field, describes resiliency as being that which produces the capacity to become competent and goal directed, allowing individuals to right themselves when the environment produces a good many awful conditions. She explains that resiliency is not a trait for a gifted few people. It is a universal genetic trait, meaning that every individual is born with resiliency.

Benard says that three categories of protective factors help individuals reshape devastating events and develop strength or resiliency. The first factor is *caring relationships,* which convey safety and basic trust. For example, the cordons of parents lining the walkways when students at Colorado's Columbine High School returned to their building in the fall of 1999 were symbols of safety and trust.

> The second factor is high expectations, ones that communicate firmness and look for strength, rather that deficits, in adolescents.

The second factor is *high expectations,* ones that communicate firmness and look for strength, rather that deficits, in adolescents. *Healthy Teens* reminds parents and caregivers to say "I love you; I expect you home at 11:00 p.m. without fail;" or "I know you want to be an engineer and you will keep your grades up;" or "I have zero tolerance for alcohol or any substance use in this family."

The third factor that builds resiliency is that of *contributing to the community.* For example, if your teen loves animals, a volunteer job in an animal shelter may be a positive way to participate in the community. If your family is politically active, he or she can explore campaigning for the governor, mayor, or sheriff. If a friend has diabetes, HIV or cancer, your adolescent can begin to help by working on marches to raise money. Stories of how young people make a difference in society are far more numerous than the newspapers have space to print.

Steven J. Wolin, M.D., and Sybil Wolin, Ph.D., other eminent researchers, define resilience as the process of bouncing back from adversity. They warn us not to believe that there are "super kids" able to endure hardships and come out completely unscathed. They do not care for the "at risk" concept that places emphasis on the vulnerability and deficits of youngsters who have met adversity. Rather, they see psychological damages but also enduring strength from struggling with hardship.

The Wolins use the word "resiliencies" to describe clusters of strength that are energized in the struggle with hardship. The seven clusters are:

- INSIGHT: The habit of asking tough questions and giving honest answers.
- INDEPENDENCE: Emotional and physical distancing from the source of troubles in one's life.
- RELATIONSHIPS: Intimate and fulfilling ties to others.
- INITIATIVE: A push for mastery.
- CREATIVITY: Self-expression through art forms.
- HUMOR: Finding the comic in the tragic.
- MORALITY: The activity of an informed conscience.

The Wolins regard the seven resiliencies as tools to be used by teachers, clinicians, and prevention workers. They serve as a mental map to help professionals know where to look for strengths in the stories of youth that are laden with problems and seemingly insurmountable obstacles. We suggest these resiliencies to parents and caregivers believing that those closest to young people will value the insights offered.

Each of the resiliencies is described and illustrated in the Wolins' book *The Resilient Self: How Survivors of Troubled Families Rise Above Adversity.* Young people talk about each of the resiliencies in their video *Survivor's Pride: Building Resilience in Youth at Risk.* Dr. Sybil Wolin, with co-author Youth Communication, has a forthcoming book (2000) *The Struggle to be Strong.*

PROGRAMMING FOR HEALTHY TEENS

The encouraging news for the future is that there have emerged a good number of models that parents and professionals can draw upon to build on the strengths of their young people. These include those from the National Youth Network from the U.S. Department of Justice, and their helpful *Youth in Action* newsletters. The National Youth Network, a part of the Department of Justice, consists of diverse youth leaders from across the nation—with the goal of uniting youth to have impact on communities throughout our nation.

In a similar way, judges and trial courts are adopting a new problem-solving orientation to their work well removed from the stereotype of the cold, disinterested magistrate. Refer to the REFERENCES AND RESOURCES section for a review of a late 1999 video *Juvenile Court: A Reality Check* produced in Oakland County, Michigan, that brilliantly illustrates a caring juvenile justice system.

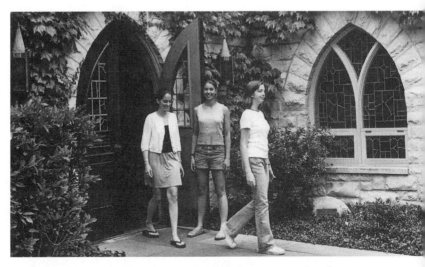

Faith communities offer many opportunities for young people to become involved in positive activities, including service to the larger community.

Schools, faith communities, Boys and Girls Cubs of America, 4-H Programs, Girl Scouts, Boy Scouts, Big Brothers, and Big Sisters are some of the community focus points that promote mentoring and tutoring opportunities, peer relationships, recreational programs, volunteering opportunities to share skills and knowledge, and community service projects. Please check the REFERENCES AND RESOURCES section for more programs and ideas to build community support for healthy adolescent development. The following two sections of this chapter describe two prevention-based programs that are being broadly used in this country.

COMMUNITIES THAT CARE

Over 500 communities across the United States have accessed the services of a nationwide system of services called Communities That Care (CTC). CTC is a system of programs and services designed to promote the healthy development of children and youth in local communities. All of the work of CTC is based on the latest research available, yet the programs are targeted for use in everyday community settings through books, teaching manuals, planning kits, youth survey information, newsletters, and consultation for training and technical assistance. CTC uses a prevention-based approach to predict and target early factors that lead to adolescent problem behaviors such as substance abuse, delinquency, teen pregnancy, school dropout and violence.

The CTC program serves as a good example of a community-based program that understands the combined strength that results from involving people from many different, overlapping parts of the community to promote the health of youth—parents, youth, elected key leaders, law enforcement, schools, local youth and family service agencies and organizations, area faith communities, the business community, and residents. The program demonstrates this same approach by gathering its research from a variety of fields, including sociology, psychology, education, public health, criminology, medicine, and organizational development.

CTC is designed to be adapted to the individual needs of each particular community, rather than taking a one-solution-fits-all approach to prevention program use. For instance, if a community has an existing mentoring program and the community members want to be sure that it is an effective program for reducing risk behaviors, they could use the information given by CTC that explains the specific components that make mentoring programs effective and apply them to their existing program. As another example, CTC consultants can advise a community on how to use its own local data as a database to generate long-range prevention planning strategies tailored for its own strengths, gaps, and needs.

A number of states have adopted CTC as their statewide model for prevention of one or more adolescent problem behaviors. The REFERENCES AND RESOURCES section of this chapter provides full contact information for this system of services.

THE SEARCH INSTITUTE

The Search Institute, located in Minneapolis, Minnesota, suggests that the real challenge in America is much deeper than acquiring a positive attitude. They say parents and adult community members must rebuild the developmental infrastructure for our children and adolescents. Please see the REFERENCES AND RESOURCES section for several references to the Search Institute.

The Power of Assets

The Search Institute has created a model for understanding the developmental needs of children and adolescents by studying more than 250,000 youth in grades six to 12. Their framework identifies 40 building blocks or "developmental assets," that all children and adolescents need to grow up healthy, competent and caring. These assets provide a powerful paradigm for mobilizing communities, organizations and individuals to take action for youth—action that can make a real difference.

Assets include family support, a caring neighborhood, parental involvement in schooling, positive peer influence, school boundaries with clear rules and consequences, a commitment to learning, positive values, skills in resisting negative peer pressure and ways to build positive self esteem. Students with high assets are more likely to resist sexual experimentation, refuse to use drugs and maintain good health. They will grow up to be caring, competent individuals.

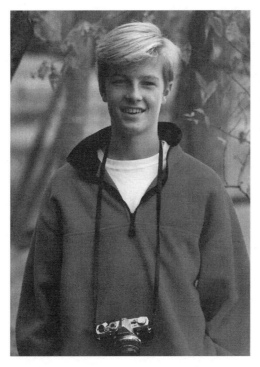

This is Michael McCarthy, age 15, the photographer for selected photos in Healthy Teens. *It is very important for adults to utilize the talents of all young people in meaningful work and volunteer service.*

The Healthy Community

For several decades, Americans have invested tremendous time, energy and resources in trying to combat drug abuse, teen pregnancy and other breakdowns in morals. Although some progress has been made, a sweeping approach is needed, one that focuses energy, creativity, and resources into rebuilding the development foundation for all youth.

As we begin to shift our thinking, we can anticipate creating communities where all young people are valued and valuable, problems more manageable, and where an attitude of vision, hope and celebration permeates community life.

Based on literature, research and work with numerous communities, the Search Institute developed a list of key characteristics of healthy communities. This includes:

Community Mindset:
- Children and youth are a top priority.
- All citizens have responsibility for children and youth.
- All citizens have pro-child power.
- The community understands that all children need more assets.
- Emphasis is placed on building family strengths.
- The community "wraps its arms" around teenagers.
- The community balances prevention and promotion.

Community Data:
- The community gathers good data on pro-child resources, programs and strategies.
- The community understands levels of assets and at-risk behaviors in its own youth, and monitors changes in assets and at-risk behaviors.

Community Norms:
- The community shares and demonstrates in concrete ways basic values such as responsibility, respect, honesty, justice and equality.
- The community demonstrates clear and consistent policies on alcohol and other drugs. Policies are consistently and actively put into practice.

Community Programming:
- After-school care is available for all children and youth.
- A rich variety of school-based, community, and religious organizations involve youth in constructive activities.

- Organizations have expansive missions that include both prevention and promotion.
- Youth programs operate with a partnership mentality.
- Programs reinforce each other appropriately.
- Peers educate and support each other.
- Mentoring is widespread (youth to youth and adult to youth).
- Young people are involved in and empowered through community service.

Community Education:

- Parent education is available, and parents participate in it.
- Adult volunteers receive training and continuing education.
- Schools are caring and supportive for youth.

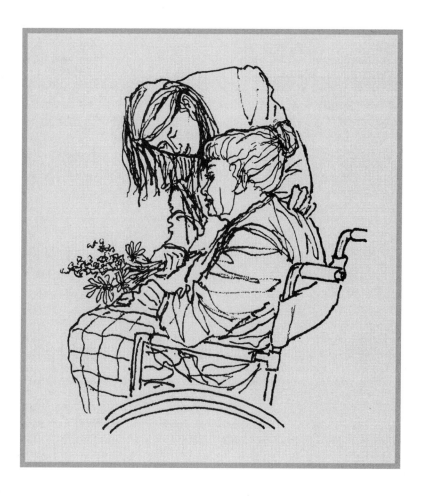

REFERENCES AND RESOURCES R/R

Beyond Leaf Raking: Learning to Serve/Serving to Learn, Peter L. Benson and Eugene C. Roehlkepartain (Abingdon Press, 1993, $14.95). Youth who serve others are more likely to have a positive outlook on life, and are far less likely than other youth to be involved in at-risk behaviors. Practical checklists, worksheets, and surveys included.

Building Business Support for School Health Programs: An Action Guide, Carlos A. Vega-Matos, Project Director (National Association of State Boards of Education, 277 South Washington Street, Suite 100, Alexandria VA 22314, 703-684-4000, E-mail address: boards@nasbe.org, Web site: www.nasbe.org., 1999, $29.00). This guide was developed to help state and local coalitions communicate effectively with the public about how coordinated school health programs help improve students' health and academic performance. Included in the guide is a set of template materials and communication tools to help users in their outreach efforts. The guide includes a CD-ROM that can be used by both Macintosh and PC-based computers.

Catch the Spirit: A Student's guide to Community Service (Prudential in cooperation with the United States Department of Education. Consumer Information Center, Department 506E, Pueblo, CO 81009, free.)

The Coalition for America's Children (888-544-KIDS, Web site: www.usakids.org.) The Benton Foundation is a founding member of the Coalition for America's Children and has supported its development as the public education arm of the children's movement. This nonprofit group links more than 450 nonprofit groups that campaign for kids under the banner "Who's for Kids—and Who's Just Kidding," providing voter education materials to help citizens prioritize children's issues.

Communities that Care (Developmental Research and Programs, 1230 Nickerson Street, Suite 107, Seattle, WA 98109, 800-736-2630, E-mail address: info@drp.org, Web site: www.drp.org.) CTC is a community operating system with researched-based tools to help communities promote the positive development of children and youth, and prevent adolescent substance abuse, delinquency, school dropout, teen pregnancy, and violence. These tools include training and technical assistance, a CTC Community Planning Kit, Prevention Strategies: A Research Guide to What Works!, and the CTC Youth Survey for measuring youth problem behaviors.

The Condition of Education 1998 (U.S. Department of Education, 877-433-7827, request report #NCES98-018). A compendium of educational statistics, including extensive information on volunteer activities. It suggests that schools shouldn't force students to volunteer, that the key to kindling a community spirit is to make a variety of activities available.

Connect for Kids (The Benton Foundation, 1634 Eye Street NW, 11th Floor, Washington DC 20006, fax-202-638-5771, Web site: www.connectforkids.org.) A virtual encyclopedia of information for adults who want to make their communities better places for kids. Their award-winning Web site, e-mail newsletters, radio, print and TV ads help people become more active citizens—from volunteering to voting. The *Connect for Kids Help Wanted Ads,* developed by children's advocacy and service groups, offer hundreds of ways to use skills, interests, and experience to help kids in cities throughout the U.S. The *Connect for Kids* team is made up of children's experts, journalists, and communications specialists in Washington, DC.

Independent Sector. (1200 Eighteenth Street NW, Suite 200, Washington DC 20036, 202-467-6100, fax-202-467-6101. E-mail Address: info@indepsec.org, Web site: www.indepsec.org.) A membership organization that brings together foundations, non-profit groups and corporate giving programs to support philanthropy, volunteering, and citizen action. Web site includes *Give Five Program*. The message of *Give Five* is to thank the majority of Americans who already give time or money, and to encourage everyone to imagine what their community would be like if everyone gave more. This program offers on-line tips on deciding where to volunteer, making the most out of volunteering experience, and links to useful volunteering sites.

Juvenile Court: A Reality Check, Citizen's Alliance of the Oakland County Probate Court and Circuit Court-Family Division (Contact Karen MacKenzie, Resource and Program specialist, Oakland County Circuit Court-Family Division, 1200 N. Telegraph, Pontiac 48341-0449, 248-858-0053, 1999, $20.00). The video depicts the experiences of three juveniles as they enter the court system and encounter the consequences for their criminal acts. Children and parents are typically confused and anxious about the juvenile court process and the services provided. This video is an attempt to realistically portray how the court works to hold youth accountable for their crimes. Highly recommended.

The Kid's Guide to Service Projects: Over 500 Service Ideas for Young People Who Want to Make a Difference, Barbara A. Lewis (Free Spirit Publishing, 1995, $10.95). This guide has something for everyone who wants to make a difference, from simple projects to large-scale commitments. Kids can choose from a variety of topics, including animals, crime fighting, the environment, friendship, hunger, literacy, politics and government, and transformation.

Resiliency in Action (P.O. Box 684, Gorham ME 04038, 800-440-5171, fax-207-839-6379, E-mail Address: nanh@connectnet.com, Web site: www.resiliency.com.) *Resiliency in Action* is a journal dedicated to the exciting, hopeful, and very real concept of resiliency. Evidence is all around of the ability of children, youth, adults, organizations, and communities to bounce back from stress and adversity. The journal's purpose is to spread the news of resiliency through sharing research and facilitating the practical application and evaluation of the resiliency paradigm. Also offering a new book put together from the first two years of the journal, *Resiliency In Action: Practical Ideas for Overcoming Risks and Building Strengths in Youth, Families, and Communities* is filled with information you need to know to move your family, your school, your community, and children and youth whom you work with from risk to resiliency.

The Resilient Self: How Survivors of Troubled Families Rise Above Adversity, Steven J. Wolin and Sybil Wolin (Villard Books, 1993, $23.00). The authors, a clinical professor of psychiatry and a developmental psychologist, point out to victims and therapists alike that children of troubled families may be more instrumental in their own survival than they realize. This is a self-help volume for adult children of dysfunctional families that puts the emphasis on rising above adversity rather than on reliving the pain of abusive relationships. The authors are co-founders of a national initiative called *Project Resilience*. For information on *Project Resilience*, the video *Survivor's Pride: Building Resilience in Youth at Risk*, and the forthcoming book *The Struggle to be Strong*, contact: Project Resilience, 5410 Connecticut Avenue, NW, Suite 113, Washington DC 20015, 202-966-8171, fax-202-966-7587, E-mail address: info@projectresilience.com, Web site: www.projectresilience.com.

School-Based Prevention for Children at Risk: The Primary Mental Health Project, Emory L. Cowen, Ed. (American Psychological Association, Web site: www.apa.org/books/school.html, $29.95, 1996). This book describes the daily operation of the Primary Mental Health Project (PMHP), an innovative school-based prevention program that provides an alternative to "after-the-fact" treatment and intervention. This book provides the tools for implementing and evaluating the PMHP, as well as research documenting the program's efficacy. The program has been in existence for over forty years and is operating in over 700 schools.

The Search Institute (700 South Third Street, Suite 210, Minneapolis, MN 55415, 800-888-7828, E-mail address: si@search-institute.org, Website: www.search-institute.org.) An independent, nonprofit organization committed to contributing to the knowledge base about youth development, and also committed to translating high-quality research on children and youth into practical ideas, tools, services, and resources for families, neighborhoods, schools, organizations, and communities. SI cites 40 assets which build character and reliability in youth. They publish studies, newsletters, and a variety of information.

Therapeutic Jurisprudence and the Emergence of Problem-Solving Courts, David Rottman and Pamela Casey in *National Institute of Justice Journal*, July 1999. This article describes how individual judges, trial courts, and entire State court systems are adopting a new, problem-solving orientation to their work, a move away from the stereotype of a cold, disinterested judge.

What Do You Stand For?: A Kids Guide to Building Character, Barbara A. Lewis (Free Spirit, 1997, $18.95). Be sure the adolescent in your home has a chance to read this outstanding book. As the author says, "The goal of this book is to help you understand yourself better, figure out what you stand for, and what you won't stand for." Wonderfully written with lots of positive examples of character building in action. The book includes actual photos of adolescents who care, respect life, are honest, responsible, and have courage.

What Kids Need to Succeed: Proven, Practical Ways to Raise Good Kids, Peter L. Benson, Judy Galbraith, and Pamela Espeland (Free Spirit Pub, 1998, $5.99). Kids who build assets and connections with home and community have more of a chance to succeed in later in life than those whose parents indulge them and try to provide the assets themselves: this is the message of a strong title encouraging parents to work with the community. More than 500 common-sense ideas for building assets in youth.

Who Cares Magazine (1436 U Street NW #201, Washington DC 20009, 202-588-8920, fax-202-986-3944, E-mail Address: info@whocares.org, Web site: www.whocares.org.) This is a magazine for innovators in social change organizations. It chronicles the youth-service movement and includes a resource directory of innovative, youth-led programs around the country.

Women's Educational Equity Act (WEEA) Equity Resources Center (Education Development Center, Inc., 800-225-3088, Web site: www.edc.org/WomensEquity). 1999 catalog of gender-fair educational resources is available. The catalog covers topics ranging from a middle and high school multicultural women's history curriculum to a working paper that helps teachers, administrators, and researchers look at the role gender plays in the application of technology. More than 100 curriculums, activity kits, working papers, and digests cover issues including gender equity, disabilities, history, life skills training, professional development, school and community safety, and school-to-work.

Worth the Risk: True Stories About Risk Takers Plus How You Can Be One, Too, Arlene Erlbach (Free Spirit, 1998, $12.95). In this examination of the value of taking risks, the true-life case studies of 20 teenagers are presented, along with information on how to go about taking a risk. The book looks at the difference between positive and negative risks, helps kids weigh the consequences, and gives advice on how to successfully execute a risk-taking plan and what to do in case of disappointment.

Your Time-Their Future is a national public education campaign developed by the U.S. Department of Health and Human Services. The campaign encourages adults to become involved in volunteering, mentoring, and other efforts that help young people ages 7 to 14 participate in positive activities that build skills, self-discipline, and competence. Web site: www.health.org/yourtime.

Youth as Resources (1700 K St. N.W., Washington D.C. 20006-3817, 202-466-6272). This program encourages youth involvement by awarding small grants to youth-run community projects.

APPENDIX I - A LOAD OFF THE TEACHERS' BACKS: COORDINATED SCHOOL HEALTH PROGRAMS

The following is an excerpt from a Kappan Special Report written by Harriet Tyson in *Phi Delta Kappan*, January 1999, pp. K2-K4.

The Poor Health of American Children

The traditional diseases of childhood have nearly disappeared, thanks to great advances in medical research and the managerial brilliance of the public health apparatus in the United States. But new health problems have emerged with a vengeance. One child in four—fully 10 million—is at risk of failure in school because of social, emotional, and health handicaps.[1]

The "new morbidities," as they are called in the public health community, are the adverse consequences of poor nutrition, lack of exercise, smoking, early sexual activity, drinking, drug abuse, violence, depression, and stress. The origins are psychological and social, but the consequences are medical, educational, and sometimes criminal: HIV/AIDS, other sexually transmitted diseases, teen pregnancy, alcohol-related automobile accidents, addiction, injuries or deaths from stabbings or shootings, and suicide.

A quick rundown of the incidence of risky behaviors among young people gives a snapshot of the problems of students in grades 9 through 12. Consider the following items, taken, unless otherwise noted, from the 1997 Youth Risk Behavior Survey (YRBS) conducted by the U.S. Centers for Disease Control and Prevention:

- 73% of all deaths among youth and young adults (10 to 24 years of age) result from only four causes: motor vehicle crashes, other unintentional injuries, homicide, and suicide.
- 19.3% of adolescents had rarely or never worn a seat belt.
- 36.6% had ridden with a driver who had been drinking alcohol.
- 50.8% had drunk alcohol during the 30 days preceding the survey, and 31.1% had first drunk alcohol before the age of 13.
- 26.2% had used marijuana during the 30 days preceding the survey.
- 7.7% had attempted suicide during the 12 months prior to the survey.
- 36% of high school students had smoked cigarettes during the 30 days prior to the survey.
- 70.7% had not eaten five or more servings of fruits and vegetables during the day preceding the survey.
- 72.6% had not attended physical education classes daily.
- 67% of all deaths and morbidities among adults under 25 years of age are the result of just two causes: cardiovascular disease and cancer,

largely attributable to poor health habits initiated during adolescence.

- HIV is increasing disproportionately among black and Hispanic young people, especially females. Although there is a trend toward more responsible behavior (less sexual activity, fewer partners, more condom use), it won't be known for some years whether these trends will result in fewer cases.[2] As matters stand, about three million teenagers contract sexually transmitted diseases annually.
- Rates of teen pregnancies in the U.S. have been declining for the past several years, but they are still the highest among industrialized nations. About a million teens become pregnant each year.[3]
- The number of teachers reporting disruptive student behavior in class is at an all-time high (47%).[4]
- Weapon violence, despite the recent rash of shootings, is declining, but only slightly. In 1997, 12.5% of males and 3.7% of females said they had carried a weapon on school property on one or more days during the 30 days prior to the survey.
- Fistfights in school are very common. Nationwide, 14.8% of students had been in a physical fight on school property one or more times during the 12 months preceding the survey.

Children who are aggressive and disruptive in the early grades are very likely to become involved in several of the "new morbidities." Children who do not learn to read in the first few grades, who read poorly, or who are retained in grade more than once are far more likely than their peers to be drawn into a pattern of risky behaviors. Thirty-five percent of students who don't read well will drop out of high school.[5] Sixty percent of adolescents in treatment for substance abuse have learning disabilities.[6] Half of juvenile delinquents tested were found to have undetected learning disabilities.[7] Among the children classified with "learning disabilities," 75% to 80% are of average or above-average intelligence and still have significant reading disabilities, according to the National Institutes of Health.

Physical inactivity is now widespread among American students. The 1997 YRBS shows that 63.8% of students nationwide had engaged in activities that made them sweat and breathe hard for at least 20 minutes on three or more of the seven previous days. The remaining 36.2% are sedentary youngsters prone to the same health risks as sedentary adults.

In addition, the eating habits of American children are poor and grow worse as they advance through the grades. The immediate consequences of eating too much salt, fat, and sugar and too few fruits, vegetables, and grains are obesity, high blood pressure, juvenile diabetes, and high rates of dental caries. Poor eating habits laid down in childhood are desperately hard to break, as every dieting adult knows.

Asthma has reached near-epidemic levels, although there is not yet a national asthma registry. The incidence is higher in the cities than in the suburbs, but even some suburban jurisdictions report that asthma is the leading cause of school absences, emergency room visits, and hospital admissions.

Finally, environmentally caused illnesses are on the rise among children and adults who work in school buildings. Children are more susceptible to environmental hazards than adults, and those hazards are increasing in numbers and intensity, both in and out of school buildings.[8] Poor indoor and outdoor air quality, contaminated water supplies, and bacterial contamination of food cause many missed school days and sometimes serious and lasting health problems.

The Poor Health of Poor Children

Children are the poorest group of Americans. What's more, they are getting poorer, and the frequencies of the contemporary health plagues are all markedly higher among children of the poor than among children of the middle class.[9] U.S. Census data show that, in 1993, 14.4% of American children were living in poverty. By 1996, the rate had risen to 20.5%. Among that group are a stunning 11.3 million American children under the age of 18 who are not covered by medical insurance. Moreover, 92.1% of uninsured children in 1996 had at least one working parent.[10] Welfare reform removed many children from Medicaid eligibility because their eligibility was contingent upon the receipt of cash benefits. The good news is that the federally sponsored Child Health Insurance Program (CHIP) promises some relief; an estimated four to five million of the 11 million uninsured children will qualify for health insurance under CHIP when it is fully implemented.

We Have Been Here Before

This is not the first time in American history that schools have been overwhelmed by a widespread crisis in child health. In the late 19th and early 20th centuries, when the last wave of immigration was in full swing, public health officials began to conduct sanitary inspections of school buildings, and cadres of nurses routinely examined school children in order to stem the tide of absences caused by the spread of infectious diseases. Health education became entrenched in the curriculum. There were crusades to stamp out tuberculosis, and the temperance movement pressed the schools to teach children about the effects of tobacco, alcohol, and narcotics on the human body. Physical education was introduced into the schools because school leaders believed it was important to health and learning. At the turn of the century, doctors removed tonsils and adenoids on school property because parents couldn't afford the carfare to the nearest dispensary.[11]

As the wave of poor immigrants subsided in the early 1900s, so did the impetus for school-based or school-linked health services. The American Medical Association (AMA) became adamant about limiting the role of school nurses and public health physicians to health screenings and restricting them from providing treatment, either on school property or at public health clinics.[12] (The AMA has changed its stance in modern times.) The wall between public health and education became higher in the middle decades of the 20th century, and their respective bureaucracies and professional cultures became more isolated from one another.

Many features of the 1990s echo those of the turn of the century: a tidal wave of immigrants, urban and rural poverty, the enduring racial divide, a lack of affordable housing and health care for the poor, and political resistance to linking education and public health. Some new elements have been added to the picture, including a drop in the age of sexual maturation, an increase in single-parent families, a reduction in the number of stay-at-home mothers, the emergence of HIV, the appearance of new and more addictive drugs, the increased availability of firearms, and skyrocketing medical costs.

The features of the 1990s, both old and new, constitute risk factors for young people and directly affect their health and well-being. And their impact is not limited to those who are poor. In virtually all school communities, the problems that contribute to the new morbidities and mortalities are present. Children in all circumstances are affected by the stresses of divorce and immigration, and adolescents everywhere are vulnerable to sexual temptation, alcohol, drugs, tobacco, depression, suicide, and violence.

A Solution: The Coordinated School Health Initiative

The coordinated school health initiative has emerged in response to the state of affairs in children's health and education today. It follows decades of mutual disengagement between the schools and community programs for public and private health, mental health, dental health, social services, recreation, and youth development. This disengagement has led to wasteful duplication of services, a jumble of separately funded prevention programs, and a widespread failure to integrate services essential to children's health and learning. The movement to provide coordinated school health services engages all the centers of activity—in and out of school—that relate to student health and success in school. It determines what the health problems are in particular school communities, builds community consensus on what services should be provided, melds funding from a variety of existing sources, and knits together a coherent and comprehensive approach that can make a difference in improving children's health.

Uncoordinated school health programs. Examples of an uncoordinated approach to student health can be observed in many schools. Lack of coordination is so normal that many school people accept fragmentation, duplication, and inconsistency as a fact of life. Examples abound.

- A depressed, pregnant, drug-using teenager in Maryland saw three counselors each week — a suicide prevention counselor, a parenting counselor, and a drug abuse counselor — and none of them talked to the others. All the while, the student missed so many classes that she flunked the semester and dropped out when her baby was born.
- While a Virginia teacher taught the children about the food pyramid, the cafeteria manager prepared a lunch of pizza and french fries, the school business manager counted the proceeds from the soft drink

and candy machines, and a nurse counseled a group of obese girls.

- Students whose immunizations are incomplete when they enroll in a new school often find themselves barred from school for a period of time while their immunizations are completed. In a large Maryland school district, a child may miss the first critical weeks of school because the public health clinic conducts immunizations on Mondays and Thursdays during business hours, and many parents cannot take a day off from work without losing their jobs or can't get to the clinic because it isn't on a bus route.
- The health education curriculum presents information about the dangers of smoking, but school policy allows students to smoke on the playground.
- Nobody asks the custodian or the secretary (both of whom probably know more about what the troubled kids are up to than anyone else in the building) to share their observations about kids.
- One-shot teacher workshops abound. They are intended to change teachers' instructional practices or their attitudes toward students, but research studies show that they have little or no effect.[13]
- A Washington, D.C., teacher emphasizes the importance of washing hands, but only one out of eight faucets in the girls' lavatory yields any water, and the maintenance department hasn't scheduled plumbing renovations for another two years.

These examples of poor communication, mixed messages, lopsidedness, wasted motion, counterproductive moves, and missed opportunities are the ground from which coordinated school health programs have arisen.

Coordinated school health programs. The guiding principle of the coordinated school health movement is that schools and communities can do a lot more than they now do with the money, staff, time, and creativity they have. Working in partnership with health agencies, community institutions, and families, schools and communities can create a seamless web of education and services that lowers the barriers to learning experienced by so many of today's young people.

Coordinated school health efforts reflect a state of mind. They rest on the premise that everybody in a child's environment can contribute something, while no one can address a child's health problems effectively by working alone. All players need to be able to cross disciplinary boundaries, employment categories, and social-class barriers. Providing for coordinated school health services requires a strong school leader who isn't afraid to take stands on issues that matter to children's well-being. It is also essential to have a skilled coordinator to pull all the disparate forces together and a strong school-site health team to pool knowledge, manage cases, and ensure the connections to agencies outside the school. Teacher involvement in school health teams is crucial because teachers have their fingers on the actual pulse of a school and have a sense of what kinds of arrangements will earn the trust and participation of students and families. The cost of coordinated school health programs is either nil or modest, and the payoff is large.

1. Joy G. Dryfoos, Full Service Schools: A Revolution in Health and Social Services for Children, Youth, and Families (San Francisco: Jossey-Bass, 1994).
2. Susan Okie, "AIDS Education Sessions Successful," Washington Post, 19 June 1998, p. A-3.
3. Douglas Kirby, No Easy Answer (Washington, D.C.: Task Force on Effective Programs and Research, National Campaign to Prevent Teen Pregnancy, 1997).
4. National Center for Education Statistics, U.S. Department of Education, teacher surveys of the school and staffing surveys, 1990-91 and 1993-94. Unpublished tabulations prepared by Westat, 1995.
5. "Learning Disabilities and Juvenile Justice," LDA Newsbriefs, January/February 1996, p. 21.
6. Ibid.
7. Ibid.
8. William J. Rea, "Why Children Are More Susceptible to Environmental Hazards," in Norma L. Miller, ed., The Healthy School Handbook: Conquering the Sick Building Syndrome and Other Environmental Hazards in and Around Your School (Washington, D.C.: National Education Association, 1995).
9. The State of America's Children: Yearbook 1998 (Washington, D.C.: Children's Defense Fund, 1998), p. xiv.
10. Bureau of the Census, U.S. Department of Commerce, Current Population Survey, March 1996 and 1997.
11. "Evolution of School Health Programs," in Diane Allensworth et al., eds., Schools and Health: Our Nation's Investment (Washington, D.C.: Institute of Medicine, National Academy Press, 1997).
12. Julia S. Lear, "School-Based Services and Adolescent Health: Past, Present, and Future," Adolescent Medicine: State of the Art Reviews, June 1996, pp. 163-68.
13. Thomas Corcoran, Transforming Professional Development for Teachers: A Guide for State Policymakers (Washington, D.C.: National Governors' Association, 1995); and David K. Cohen and Heather Hill, Classroom Performance: The Mathematics Reform in California (Philadelphia: Center for Policy Research in Education, University of Pennsylvania, 1998).

Reprinted with permission from the Educational Development Center, Inc. This Special Report was developed under contract with Education Development Center, Inc., Newton, Mass., with fiscal support provided by a cooperative agreement with the U.S. Centers for Disease Control and Prevention, National Center for Chronic Disease Prevention and Health Promotion, Division of Adolescent and School Health, Atlanta, Georgia. The contents of the Special Report are the responsibility of its author and do not necessarily reflect the official views of the U.S. Centers for Disease Control and Prevention. See the REFERENCES AND RESOURCES section of chapter two for a full resource listing of this report.

APPENDIX 2 - THE MICHIGAN MODEL FOR COMPREHENSIVE SCHOOL HEALTH EDUCATION

Scheduled Modules for Grades 7-12 for 1999

The skills taught in each lesson are listed following the title.

Grades 7-8

THE TWO "R'S" FOR STOPPING ASSAULT AND PREVENTING VIOLENCE (15 lessons)

- Anger management
- Negotiation
- Evaluating social influences
- Managing intimidation
- Avoiding and escaping violence
- Dealing effectively with sexual harassment and abusive relationships

This module is supplemented by three resources: one for parents, which is linked to the curriculum and includes parent group lessons, one for teachers, which addresses issues such as how and when to refer students for further assistance, and a resource to assist in the development of a comprehensive school violence prevention program.

IT'S NO MYSTERY: TOBACCO IS A KILLER (7 lessons)

- Evaluation of advertising techniques
- Counter-advertising to sell a "no use" message
- Refusal skills
- Supporting people who are abstaining or trying to quit
- Avoiding secondhand smoke

IT'S TIME TO MOVE! (4 lessons)
- Logging personal physical activity
- Examination of personal barriers to being physically active
- Development of a personal plan to be physically active

WHAT'S FOOD GOT TO DO WITH IT? (8 lessons)

- Evaluation of nutritional information on packaged food
- Counter-advertising
- Fast food survival
- Advocating for good nutrition

HIV, AIDS AND OTHER STDs (8 lessons)

- Evaluating the risks
- Adopting a plan to stay within sexual limits

- Clear communication
- Identifying trouble situations
- Avoiding and escaping risky situations
- Planning and sharing ways to be positive role models

Grades 9-12

MANAGING CONFLICTS AND PREVENTING VIOLENCE (16 lessons)

- Evaluating the impact of media on violence
- Analyzing the impact of violence on perpetrators, victims, families, friends, and communities
- Expressing emotions constructively
- Negotiating and de-escalating
- Responding constructively to the anger of others
- Developing a personal anger management plan

TEENS CAMPAIGN AGAINST TOBACCO (6 lessons)

- Preparation of an anti-tobacco campaign
- Communicating concern without alienating others
- Helping others quit

HELP YOURSELF TO GOOD NUTRITION (12 lessons)

- Applying a formula for weight management
- Preparing a healthy weight loss plan
- Formulating nutritional advice for hypothetical teens
- Identifying ways to improve the school lunch menu

STAY PHYSICALLY ACTIVE - FOR LIFE (4 lessons)

- Examining barriers to being physically active
- Developing a personal plan to be physically active
- Advocating for physical activity

Also available are middle and high school guides for integrating these modules into a comprehensive school health education program. A substance abuse prevention module is in development; additional modules will become available as funding permits. For more information and copies of the modules, contact the Educational Material Center of Central Michigan University at 800-214-8961.

Reprinted with permission from the Michigan Department of Education, School Health Programs Unit, PO Box 30008, Lansing MI 48909.

APPENDIX 3 - MAKING THE GRADE: A GUIDE TO SCHOOL DRUG PREVENTION

Nine Key Elements of Effective Drug Prevention Curricula
The Eight Top Drug Prevention Programs in the U.S.

Key Elements of Effective Drug Prevention Curricula:

Extensive research during the past two decades points to certain key elements of successful prevention curricula. Experts believe that these elements should be part of a comprehensive strategy in the school, the home and the community so that everyone who touches the life of a young person presents a consistent prevention message. Experts also believe that a comprehensive approach has additional benefits since many of the elements important to drug prevention are also critical in prevention of other high risk behaviors, involving violence, HIV/AIDS, sexually transmitted diseases, adolescent pregnancy and suicide. *Making the Grade* assesses the extent to which curricula address these key areas and whether curriculum activities promote necessary skills. The guide rates how well each curriculum:

- Helps students recognize internal pressures, like wanting to belong to the group, and external pressures, like peer attitudes and advertising, that influence them to use alcohol, tobacco and other drugs.
- Facilitates development of personal, social and refusal skills to resist these pressures.
- Teaches that using alcohol, tobacco and other drugs is not the norm among teenagers, correcting the misconception that "everyone is doing it," and promotes positive norms through bonding to school and constructive role models.
- Provides developmentally appropriate material and activities, including information about the short-term effects and long-term consequences of alcohol, tobacco and other drugs.
- Uses interactive teaching techniques, such as role plays, discussions, brainstorming and cooperative learning.
- Covers necessary prevention elements in at least eight well-designed sessions a year (with a minimum of three to five booster sessions in one or more succeeding years).
- Actively involves the family and the community, so that prevention strategies are reinforced across settings.
- Includes teacher training and support, in order to assure that curricula are delivered as intended.
- Contains material that is easy for teachers to implement and culturally relevant for students.

Eight Top Drug Prevention Programs

- Michigan Model for Comprehensive School Health
  Michigan Department of Community Health
  3423 N. Martin Luther King Blvd.
  Lansing, Mich. 48909
  517-335-8390
  Web site: www.emc.cmich.edu
  Grades K-12

- STAR/Students Taught Awareness and Resistance
  Department of Preventive Medicine
  University of Southern California
  1441 Eastlake Ave., MS-44
  Los Angeles, Calif. 90033-0800
  213-865-0325
  Grades 5-8

- Project TNT/Toward No Tobacco Use
  ETR Associates
  P.O. Box 1830
  Santa Cruz, Calif. 95061-1830
  800-321-4407
  Web site: www.etr.org
  Grades 5-9

- Project Northland
  Hazelden Publishing and Education
  P.O. Box 176
  Center City, Minn. 55012-0176
  800-328-9000
  www.hazelden.com
  Grades 6-8

- Project ALERT
  BEST Foundation
  725 S. Figueroa St.
  Suite 1615
  Los Angeles, Calif. 90017
  800-ALERT-10
  Web site: www.projectalert.best.org
  Grades 6,7 or 7,8

- Life Skills Training
  Princeton Health Press
  115 Wall Street
  Princeton, N.J. 08540

800-636-3415
Web site: www.lifeskillstraining.com
Grades 6-8 or 7-9

- Alcohol Misuse Prevention Program (Series II)
University of Michigan
Institute for Social Research
P.O. Box 1248
Ann Arbor, Mich. 48106-1248
734-647-0587
Grades 6-8

- Reconnecting Youth
National Educational Service
1252 Loesch Road
Bloomington, Ind. 47404
800-733-6786
Web site: www.nesonline.com
Grades 9-12

Reprinted with permission from Drug Strategies. See REFERENCES AND RESOURCES section of chapter seven for a full resource listing of this material.

APPENDIX 4 - WHEN YOUR ADOLESCENT IS IN TROUBLE

Despite a parent's best efforts, some young people find themselves in trouble with the law. Peer pressure, the need to assert independence, or misjudgments can place your adolescent at risk of involvement in activities that result in arrest and processing through the local juvenile justice system.

Juvenile justice systems vary widely between communities. If your child becomes involved in the juvenile justice system, your first step is to learn how the system in your area works. This knowledge will allow you to advocate for an outcome that teaches your child about the results of inappropriate behavior without hurting his or her prospects for the future.

Begin by asking the processing officer at the police station (usually an officer in the juvenile division) to explain the process to you:

- Why was my child arrested?
- Will you have to detain my child or can he or she be released in my custody?
- Will we need to post bond?
- Will my child have a record simply as a result of the arrest?
- What happens next?
- With whom should I speak to get assistance if my child is referred to juvenile court?

In many cases, particularly for minor offenses or a first-time arrest, youth will be released into their parent's custody. They also may be diverted into a community service program where they will be expected to perform volunteer service. In exchange, the charges against them will be dropped.

If your child is referred to juvenile court, however, what happens next will depend on the structure of the local system, the actions of the prosecutor's office, and the availability of diversion or treatment programs. The prosecutor and juvenile court staff can tell you what to expect from the process. (Juvenile court staff include intake or probation department staff who often conduct preliminary investigations. These investigations provide juvenile court judges with background information they use to decide on dispositions.)

You also are well advised to seek legal counsel if your child is referred to the court system. Youth of families without financial resources can request counsel from the local public defender's office. Even if you obtain a lawyer to represent your child, you should accompany your teen through all juvenile justice system processing: intake, meetings with juvenile court staff and diversionary or treatment program staff, and any court hearings.

Keep in mind that the main intent of most juvenile justice systems is to help young people redirect their lives, not simply to punish them. Still, your role in advocating for your child is crucial. There are several alternatives to a court hearing, court decision, or detention. Your child can be diverted, for example, into a treatment program. Further, when a court hearing and decision are required, courts usually view a parent's involvement in the case positively when making a decision.

Further, it often is in times of crisis that bonds between parents and adolescents are reaffirmed. At those times, youth again turn to their parents for support and protection. Troubling circumstances may present parents of adolescents with opportunities to show their love and support, to help their child obtain services to deal with specific problems, and to strengthen interpersonal connections that will benefit the family for years to come.

Reprinted with permission from *Supporting Your Adolescent: Tips for Parents*. Prepared by the National Clearinghouse on Families and Youth, 1996, U.S. Department of Health and Human Services. See the References and Resources section of chapter one for a full resource listing of this material.

Acknowledgments for Healthy Teens, Second Edition

The earlier editions of *Healthy Teens* formed a solid foundation for the third edition. The following individuals comprise the reviewers and supporters of the second edition. In demonstration of consistent support over the years, many of these people also offered their input for the development of the third edition of *Healthy Teens*. The Executive Editor extends her continued deep thanks to all of the following people:

Joyce Bertasio and Carol Sizemore, Allen Park, Michigan

Jerry Aris, M.B.A., President, Citizens Against Crime, Allen, Texas

Patsy Baker, Program Analyst, Rape Prevention and Services Program, Child & Family
 Services, Michigan Family Independence Agency, Lansing, Michigan

Laurie Bechhofer, M.P.H., Evaluation Consultant, Supervisor, Comprehensive Programs in Health &
 Childhood, Michigan Department of Education

Michael J. Bender, Principal, and the families of Allen Park High School,
 Allen Park, Michigan

Joyce Buchanan, Administrative Assistant to Dr. Lloyd D. Johnston, The University of Michigan
 Monitoring the Future Study, Survey Research Center, Ann Arbor, Michigan

Jean Chabut, M.P.H., Chief, Center for Health Promotion and Chronic Disease Prevention,
 Michigan Department of Community Health

Jan Christensen, J.D., M.S.W., Chief, Division of Violence, Injury, and Surveillance, Center for
 Health Promotion and Chronic Disease Prevention, Community Public Health Agency

Sue Coats, M.S.W., Program Director, Turning Point, Mt. Clemens, Michigan; Laura Coens,
 Director of Communications, Michigan Dyslexia Institute/Dyslexia Association of America

Willard R. Daggett, Ed.D., International Center for Leadership in Education, Inc., Schenectady,
 New York

Steven W. Enoch, Ed.D., former Superintendent of Schools, Bonsall Union School
 District, California

Pam Farlow-Wolgast, M.A., L.L.P., L.P.C., C.S.W., Staff Training and Development
 Coordinator, Common Ground, Pontiac, Michigan

Holly Fechner, J.D., Labor and Employment Attorney, Policy Office of the U.S. Department
 of Labor

Kathy Gibson, School Health Consultant, Center for School Community Outreach, Wayne County
 Regional Educational Services Agency, Wayne, Michigan

Althea Grant, M.S.W., A.C.S.W., Executive Director, Detroit Rape Crisis Center, Detroit
 Receiving Hospital

Naomi Haines Griffith, M.A., M.S.W., Executive Director, Parents and Children Together (PACT),
 Consultant, Alabama Children's Trust Fund, Decatur, Alabama

Detective Ronald Halcrow, Birmingham Police Department, Birmingham, Michigan

Ellen Hayse, M.S., Resource Coordinator, Resource Center on Sexual and Domestic Violence,
 Lansing, Michigan

John Howell, Ph.D., F/A.O.G.P.E., Director of Abrams Teaching Laboratory and Research,
 Michigan Dyslexia Institute/Dyslexia Association of America

Kay Howell, M.A., F/A.O.G.P.E., Michigan Dyslexia Institute/Dyslexia Association
    of America
Auleen Jarrett, R.N., B.S.N., President, CRIMEFREE Seminars, Inc., Livonia, Michigan
Rachel N. Kay, M.P.H., Cook County Department of Public Health, Oak Park, Illinois
Gloria Krys, M.A., C.S.W., L.P.C., Program Coordinator, Assault Crisis Center of Washtenaw
    County Community Mental Health, Ypsilanti, Michigan
Joseph Malgeri, M.S.M., Career Solutions, Troy, Michigan
The Michigan Department of State Police: Sergeant Joseph Hanley, Special Operations, Traffic
    Services Division; Lt. Dan Smith, Traffic Services Division; Sergeant Darwin A. Scott,
    Criminal Intelligence Unit, and Phyllis Good, Supervisor, Narcotics and Dangerous
    Drugs Unit, East Lansing Laboratory, East Lansing, Michigan
Katherine Miller, M.A., Prevention Section Chief, Office of Substance Abuse Services, Michigan
    Department of Community Health
Helene Mills, Ed.D., Principal, Seaholm High School, Birmingham, Michigan
James Moore, Program Director and Assistance Executive Director, American Lung Association,
    Lansing, Michigan
Patricia Morgan, R.N., M.S., Consultant for School Health Programs, School Health Unit,
    Michigan Department of Community Health, Lansing, Michigan
William T. Munsell, Director of Financial Aid, Lake Superior State University,
    Sault Ste. Marie, Michigan
Sherry Murphy, M.A., Consultant for Drug Free Schools, Oakland Schools Intermediate School
    District, Waterford, Michigan
Patricia Nichols, M.S., C.H.E.S., Supervisor, Comprehensive Programs in Health & Early
    Childhood, Michigan Department of Education
Carol Noël, Author, Communications Specialist, President, Serious Business, Inc.,
    Petoskey, Michigan
Karen Petersmarck, M.P.H., Ph.D., Consultant, Division of Violence, Injury and Surveillance,
    Center for Health Promotion and Chronic Disease Prevention, Community Public
    Health Agency
Andrea Poniers, M.S.S.W., Public health Consultant, Tobacco Section, Center for Health Promotion,
    Chronic Disease Prevention, Michigan Department of Community Health
Randall S. Pope, Chief, HIV/AIDS Prevention & Intervention, Michigan Department of
    Community Health
Lt. Mike Radzik, Washtenaw County Sheriff's Department, Ypsilanti, Michigan
David Rosen, M.D., M.P.H., C.S. Mott Children's Hospital, A. Alfred Taubman Health Care
    Center, Ann Arbor, Michigan
Eli Saltz, Ph.D., Director, The Merrill-Palmer Institute, Detroit, Michigan
Joy Schumacher, R.N., B.S.N., Oakland County Health Department AIDS Office,
    Pontiac, Michigan
Patricia Smith, M.S., Division of Violence, Injury, and Surveillance, Center for Health Promotion
    and Chronic Disease Prevention, Community Public Health Agency
Craig C. Spangler, D.D.S., Bloomfield Hills, Michigan
Stephen Spector, Ph.D., Psychologist, Beacon Hill Clinic, Birmingham, Michigan
Lou Stewart, M.A.T., L.D., Diagnostician and Educational Therapist, Birmingham, Michigan
James Stone, Guidance Counseling Department Head, Groves High School,
    Birmingham, Michigan
Donald B. Sweeney, M.A., Chief, School Health Unit, Michigan Department of
    Community Health
Betty Tableman, M.P.A., Director, Prevention Services, Michigan Department of
    Community Health

Lois Thieleke, M.S., Extension Home Economist, Michigan State University Extension, Oakland County, Michigan

Diane Trippett, M.S., R.D., Clinical Nutrition Manager, Dietetics Department, Children's Hospital of Michigan, Detroit, Michigan

Detective Sergeants Larry Ivory and Michael Oliver of the Waterford Township Police Department, Michigan

Howell Wechsler, Ed.D., M.P.H., Health Scientist, Division of Adolescent Health, Centers for Disease Control and Prevention, Atlanta, Georgia

Sis Wenger, M.A., Executive Director, National Association for Children of Alcoholics, Rockville, Maryland

Delores Wilson, Counselor, Allen Park Schools, Allen Park, Michigan

James Windell, M.A., L.L.P., Oakland Psychological Clinic, Oakland County Probate Court, Pontiac, Michigan

Joel L. Young, M.D., Medical Director, Psychiatric Evaluation and Referral Center, Crittenton Hospital, Rochester, Michigan

NOTE: The Michigan Department of Community Health and the Michigan Department of Education are located in Lansing, Michigan. Addresses and titles of those who have provided assistance in former years may have changed.

Index

Advanced Praise

Healthy Teens is useful to parents and young people because it presents frank information about growth such as at the time of puberty. It also gives clear instruction about the dangers of sexually transmitted diseases, including HIV/AIDS. Clinics and hospitals can use the book as they advise young people. The book also carefully explains the importance of education beyond high school to prepare for the new millennium.

Sylmara E. Chatman, M.D.
Medical Director, St. John Health System School-Based Health Clinics
Detroit, Michigan

No one is more deserving of our time and energy than our teenage children. To help us in our efforts is this wonderful, comprehensive guide—*Healthy Teens*. It is well written, easy to read, and accurately reflects the challenges our adolescent children face. In addition, the extensive list of resources will be a valuable guide for parents who do not know where to go for help. Do you want to build a better relationship between you and your teen? *Healthy Teens* will be a great place to start!

Barbara Flis
Parent of two adolescents
Northville, Michigan

Healthy Teens is an extraordinary reference for parents, teachers, principals—anyone concerned about adolescents. It is not preachy. In a down-to-earth, insightful, and very readable style, it asks adults to listen to important issues in teens' lives. It is apparent that the author cares deeply about young people, and its style invites teens to read the book for themselves.

Donald D. Gainey, Ed.D.
Principal, Milford High School
Milford, Massachusetts

Alice McCarthy continues to write meaningful books about the pressures and issues faced by young people today. *Healthy Teens* is a terrific resource for anyone who cares for adolescents.

Margaret Rose
Health Education Specialist
Utah State Office of Education

There is a lot of talk in society about overindulged and destructive teens, especially in the media. *Healthy Teens* puts into perspective the current environment for young people. It is not an apology for their behavior, but rather a well-researched proposal underlining the need for families and professionals to understand how adolescents need the careful attention of every one of us to help bring them into a healthy, well-adjusted adulthood. A must read!

Jean Schultz, M.S., CHES
Coordinator, Middle-Level AIDS Prevention/Comprehensive Health Project
National Middle School Association

Healthy Teens addresses the many health and social issues of what's happening in a teen's world. Within a framework of current research findings, this book provides teens, families, and professionals with information, resources, and guidance for implementing a comprehensive approach toward helping teens toward adjustment, resiliency, and wellness. Those involved with teens in the home, school, and/or community will find this reading to be relevant and practical for these times.

Paula R. Zaccone-Tzannetakis, Ed.D., CHES
Associate Professor of Educational Studies, Seton Hall University
South Orange, New Jersey

Healthy Teens: Facing the Challenges of Young Lives provides parents and caregivers with the same authoritative research about adolescents that professionals who work with teens use daily. The author reasons that clear explanations of what the social environment is like for young people today will help families make carefully considered decisions. She forcefully advocates for family understanding of youth development and for the deep involvement of families in education, especially health education. The information is straightforward. The book lists many resources for further study. The well-illustrated and careful design of this book will appeal to both parents and the professionals who work with adolescents.

Dorothy Beardmore
President, State Board of Education, Michigan
National Association of State Boards of Education Healthy Schools Network

ABOUT THE AUTHOR

Alice R. McCarthy, Ph.D., is a nationally known civic leader, educator, and writer. She carries degrees from Cornell University in human ecology and education. Her doctoral work in education (Wayne State University, 1986) strengthened her expertise in human growth and development across the life span, adult learning, and curriculum development.

Dr. McCarthy founded Bridge Communications, Inc., in 1987, a communications company whose mission is to provide well-researched yet readable parenting and health-related publication materials. Serving as President, she combines her skills as a researcher, writer, editor, and publisher to provide print materials, curricula, and research studies for parents and professionals across the nation. Over the years, she has assumed major community service leadership roles in three universities, and in many national, state, and local organizations. Many honors have been received for this service.

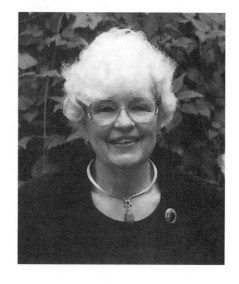

The author has a diverse array of award-winning publications and curricula to her credit. The previous two editions of *Healthy Teens*, published in 1996 and 1997, sold out within months. Her *Healthy Newsletters* are a series of four-color, four-page newsletters for families of K-3, 4-5, and 6-8 graders, with a 1.2 million annual reader base. These newsletters have won many national awards. *Health 'n Me!* is a national curriculum in health for grades K-6, brimming with well-chosen and interactive materials. In 1998, she carefully selected and annotated 300 family-oriented print and multimedia materials to provide guidance for families in site-based libraries for a major national industry. Her ongoing research concerns the needs of adults for parenting education and health education, and the status of health teaching in schools.

Dr. McCarthy brings much personal experience to her work, as a mother of five adult children and nine grandchildren. The author resides in Birmingham, Michigan, outside of Detroit, which has been home for nearly fifty years. Her gardens have been enjoyed by many. In the year 2000, she will be listed in *The Garden Conservancy: The Guide to Visiting America's Very Best Private Gardens*, and will open her lovely gardens for the public.

Caring families, friends, and supportive institutions together,
bring strength to guide adolescents toward adulthood.

Photo: Michael E. McCarthy, Age 15

This book was designed and produced in QuarkXpress on a Power Macintosh. Typeface families used throughout book are Garamond and Gill Sans. Book printing by Malloy Lithographing, Inc. Ann Arbor, MI, USA.